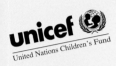
United Nations Children's Fund

WORLD HEALTH
ORGANIZATION

United Nations
Population Fund

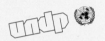

UNAIDS
UNICEF • UNDP • UNFPA • UNDCP
ILO•UNESCO•WHO•WORLD BANK

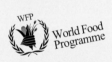
WFP
World Food
Programme

THE WORLD BANK

Factsfor Life

Third Edition

FactsforLife

Contents

The
*Facts
for Life*
topics:

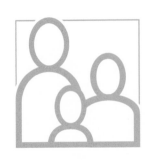

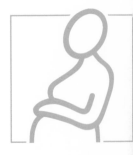

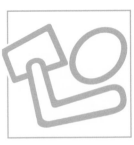

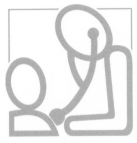

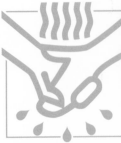

9

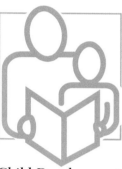
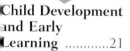

Child Development and Early Learning 21

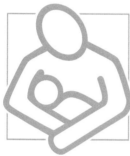

Breastfeeding 39

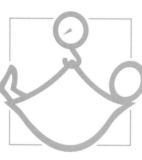

Nutrition and Growth 53

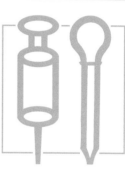

Immunization 65

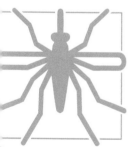

Malaria 105

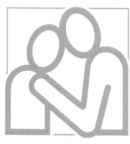

HIV/AIDS 113

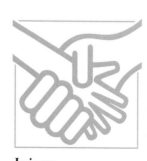

Injury Prevention........129

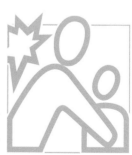

Disasters and Emergencies 143

Foreword

Every year, nearly 11 million children die from preventable causes before reaching their fifth birthday, many of them during the first year of life. Millions more survive only to face diminished lives, unable to develop to their full potential.

This terrible toll in human suffering and forgone prosperity can be vastly reduced. Three fourths of all child visits to health facilities for medical care and 7 out of 10 childhood deaths result from just five causes: pneumonia, diarrhoea, measles, malaria and malnutrition. The knowledge and capacity to prevent and treat all five causes exist.

Facts for Life aims to make life-saving knowledge easily available to everyone. It presents the most important facts that people have a right to know to prevent child deaths and diseases, and to protect women during pregnancy and childbirth. Its messages are simple, and people in every corner of the world can act on them.

Published by UNICEF, WHO, UNESCO, UNFPA, UNDP, UNAIDS, WFP and the World Bank, *Facts for Life* can save many lives – if its messages reach their intended audience. We urge all communicators – health workers, the media, government officials, non-governmental organizations, teachers, religious leaders, employers, trade unions, women's groups, community organizations and others – to join in a common cause to protect all children.

Carol Bellamy
Executive Director
United Nations Children's Fund

Dr. Gro Harlem Brundtland
Director-General
World Health Organization

Koichiro Matsuura
Director-General
United Nations Educational,
Scientific and Cultural Organization

Thoraya Ahmed Obaid
Executive Director
United Nations Population Fund

Mark Malloch Brown
Administrator
United Nations Development Programme

Dr. Peter Piot
Executive Director
Joint United Nations Programme
on HIV/AIDS

Catherine Bertini
Executive Director
World Food Programme

James D. Wolfensohn
President
The World Bank

The purpose of *Facts for Life*

Facts for Life aims to provide parents and other caregivers with the information they need to save and improve children's lives. The challenge is to ensure that everyone **knows and understands** these facts and is motivated to **put them into practice**.

The messages contained in *Facts for Life* are based on the latest scientific findings, as established by medical experts around the world. These facts are presented in non-technical language so they can be understood and acted upon easily by people who do not have a scientific background. Doing so can save lives.

Everyone can help communicate the *Facts for Life* messages – health workers, teachers, students, government officials, radio broadcasters, journalists, community workers, religious leaders and people in all walks of life – young and old, family members, friends and neighbours, men, women and children.

The structure of *Facts for Life*

Facts for Life consists of 13 chapters, each dealing with one major cause of childhood illness and death. Every chapter has three parts: an introduction, several key messages and supporting information.

The introduction is a brief and powerful 'call to action'. It summarizes the extent of the problem and why taking action is so important. The introduction aims to inspire people to get involved and share the information widely. The introduction can be used to motivate political leaders and the mass media.

The key messages, addressed to parents and other caregivers, are the essence of *Facts for Life*. They contain the essential information that people need to protect their children. The key messages are clear, brief and practical, so people can easily understand them and take the recommended action. These messages are meant to be communicated often and in various ways.

The supporting information elaborates on the key messages, providing additional details and advice. This information is particularly useful for health workers or anyone who wants to know more. It can also be used to answer caregivers' questions.

Essential *Facts*

The following are the essential messages distilled from *Facts for Life*.

1 The health of both women and children can be significantly improved when births are spaced at least two years apart, when pregnancy is avoided before age 18 and after age 35, and when a woman has no more than four pregnancies in total.

2 All pregnant women should visit a health worker for prenatal care, and all births should be assisted by a skilled birth attendant. All pregnant women and their families need to know the warning signs of problems during pregnancy and have plans for obtaining immediate skilled help if problems arise.

3 Children learn from the moment of birth. They grow and learn fastest when they receive attention, affection and stimulation, in addition to good nutrition and proper health care. Encouraging children to observe and to express themselves, to play and explore, helps them learn and develop socially, physically and intellectually.

4 Breastmilk *alone* is the only food and drink an infant needs for the first six months. After six months, infants need other foods in addition to breastmilk.

5 Poor nutrition during the mother's pregnancy or during the child's first two years can slow a child's mental and physical development for life. From birth to age two, children should be weighed every month. If a young child does not gain weight over a two-month period, something is wrong.

6 Every child needs a series of immunizations during the first year of life to protect against diseases that can cause poor growth, disability or death. Every woman of childbearing age needs to be protected against tetanus. Even if the woman was immunized earlier, she needs to check with a health worker.

7 A child with diarrhoea needs to drink plenty of the right liquids – breastmilk, fruit juice or oral rehydration salts (ORS). If the diarrhoea is bloody or

for Life messages

frequent and watery, the child is in danger and should be taken to a health centre for immediate treatment.

8 Most children with coughs or colds will get better on their own. But if a child with a cough is breathing rapidly or with difficulty, the child is in danger and needs to be taken to a health centre for immediate treatment.

9 Many illnesses can be prevented by good hygiene practices – using clean toilets or latrines, washing hands with soap and water or ash and water after defecating and before handling food, using water from a safe source, and keeping food and water clean.

10 Malaria, which is transmitted through mosquito bites, can be fatal. Wherever malaria is common, mosquito nets treated with a recommended insecticide should be used, any child with a fever should be examined by a trained health worker, and pregnant women should take antimalarial tablets recommended by a health worker.

11 AIDS is a fatal but preventable disease. HIV, the virus that causes AIDS, spreads through unprotected sex (intercourse without a condom), transfusions of unscreened blood, contaminated needles and syringes (most often those used for injecting drugs), and from an infected woman to her child during pregnancy, childbirth or breastfeeding. It is essential for everyone to know about HIV/AIDS and how to prevent it. The risk of infection through the primary sexual route can be reduced by practicing safer sex. Women who are or could be infected with HIV should consult a qualified health worker for information, counselling and testing to protect their health and reduce the risk of infecting their infants.

12 Many serious accidents can be prevented if parents or caretakers watch young children carefully and keep their environment safe.

13 In disaster or emergency situations, children should receive essential health care, including measles vaccination and micronutrient supplementation. In stressful situations, it is always preferable for children to be cared for by their parents or other familiar adults. Breastfeeding is particularly important at this time.

A guide for communicating
Facts for Life

Communication goes far beyond providing people with information. It involves listening to people, sharing information in interesting and accessible ways and helping them understand its relevance to their lives. Communicating Facts for Life *calls for an interactive, two-way process of sharing ideas, knowledge and opinions. This guide aims to help that process.*

Reaching the caregivers

Parents and caregivers, including older siblings and other family members, are the primary audience for *Facts for Life* information. They can be reached through a combination of interpersonal and mass media channels. Those who have an influence on people's health practices are the most effective communicators. They may be health workers, teachers, government extension workers, religious and community leaders, members of youth and women's groups and non-governmental organizations, employers and business people, members of trade unions, social workers, artists and entertainers.

Factors that influence communication

People's reactions to new information are influenced by how, where and from whom they receive it. These factors can mean the difference in whether or not people act on the information. People are more likely to trust information and act on it if:

- they hear it repeatedly from many different sources

- the person delivering it is well known and trusted

- they understand how it can help their families

- it is communicated in familiar language

- they are encouraged to discuss it and to ask questions to clarify their understanding of what needs to be done, when and why.

Translating and adapting the messages

The messages presented in the international version of *Facts for Life* need to be translated and, in many cases, adapted to local situations and customs. In doing so, it is crucial to check the adapted text with local health authorities before printing and disseminating to ensure that the messages remain technically valid.

Effective communication

There are many different ways of communicating, but whether you are working person-to-person within a community, advocating with political leaders or developing messages to be publicized in the mass media, the basic principles are the same:

- Know who needs the *Facts for Life* information and find out about their living conditions, language, customs and level of knowledge. This will help to identify the messages that are more relevant, more easily understood and more likely to be accepted and acted upon.

- When adapting or translating the messages, be sure to use simple language that people understand. Do not overload the messages with too many actions or technical details. *Keep to the verified information in* **Facts for Life**. If the messages are adapted, their accuracy should be verified.

- Make sure the audience understands the information and knows how to put it into practice. This can be done by sharing the draft messages and visual materials with parents and other caregivers in the community, asking them open-ended questions and encouraging discussion to determine whether the intended message is both clearly understood and feasible. Utilize their feedback to adjust the messages and visual aids.

- Make the message relevant to people's lives. Find ways to make *Facts for Life* messages interesting and meaningful to each community, such as by illustrating them with local examples.

- Select the communication channels and media that are most effective at reaching the target audience. Pay particular attention to existing media and use these media as much as possible. Do not rely on a single means of communication but instead use a mix of channels and media so that the audience receives the message repeatedly and in many variations. The mix may include:

  ○ **mass media,** such as radio, television, newspapers and comic books;

Communication breakdowns

Efforts to communicate health messages may not always achieve the intended results. Problems can usually be avoided if communicators first strive to understand the attitudes, beliefs and social factors that determine people's behaviour and the problems that may arise as people begin to change their behaviour.

- **The message may reach only some of the intended target audience because the communication channels were not effective.**

  Example: Using only printed materials – such as newspaper articles and leaflets – will not reach those who cannot read, and the use of radio and television will reach only those who have access to these media.

  Solution: If possible, use a combination of mass media to inform the audience and person-to-person communication to reinforce the message. Conduct participatory research to find out what communication channels are most likely to reach and have credibility with the audience.

- **People may receive the message but not understand it.**

  Example: The message may use technical terminology or be expressed in the wrong language or dialect.

  Solution: When translating or adapting the messages, use simple, non-technical language. Pre-test the messages to check if the intended audience understands them.

- **People may receive the message but misinterpret it and apply it incorrectly.**

○ **small media,** such as posters, audio cassettes, leaflets, brochures, videos, slide sets, flip charts, T-shirts, badges and loudspeaker announcements;

○ **interpersonal channels,** such as health workers, religious or community leaders, women's and youth organizations, school teachers, development workers and government officials.

● Repeat the information to reinforce it.

Example: Mothers who have been taught to use oral rehydration solution (ORS) may still use too much water, which makes the solution ineffective, or too little, making the solution potentially dangerous.

Solution: If any new skills are required, provide adequate training and follow up periodically to identify and correct any problems by offering additional support or revising the message.

● **People may receive and understand the information but not act on it because it conflicts with existing attitudes and beliefs.**

Example: Mothers who are instructed to continue feeding a child suffering from diarrhoea may not act on this information because it conflicts with a common, traditional belief that the stomach needs to 'rest' during diarrhoea.

Solution: Prepare messages that dispel harmful myths in a culturally sensitive way.

● **People may receive and understand the new information but be unable to act on it because of various reasons, such as poverty, or because basic services are not available.**

Example: Mass media campaigns can increase community demand for packets of ORS. But if the packets are too expensive or unavailable locally, the money spent on such mass campaigns is wasted.

Solution: Liaise with local health authorities before undertaking media campaigns to ensure that the recommended services or products are available and affordable.

Communicating through the mass media

Radio, newspapers and television are excellent tools for reaching large numbers of people to introduce and reinforce new information. Repetition strengthens memory, so publicizing the same message in various media helps people retain the message and encourages them to act on it. The information can be presented through interviews, news articles, discussions, radio or television drama, puppet shows, comics, jingles or songs, quizzes, contests and call-in shows.

- Newspaper and magazine articles are more effective where literacy rates are high. In areas where literacy is low, other means of reaching the target audience should be utilized. In some situations, comics and illustrations can be used to communicate with adults as well as children.

- If the messages are aired on radio or television, try to ensure that they are broadcast at a time when the target audience is listening or watching. Do not rely only on free public service announcements (PSAs) that are aired during off-peak hours. Broadcast the messages during popular programmes so that they reach a wide audience. Work with producers of radio or television programmes to integrate messages into the scripts of popular television shows or radio dramas, or contact popular disc jockeys who will agree to discuss the messages on radio call-in programmes.

- Use respected, credible media and public personalities to communicate and reinforce messages in the media programmes.

Communicating person-to-person

Most people are not comfortable using new information that they have learned through the media unless they have an opportunity to discuss it with someone they trust. For that reason, it is most effective to use both mass media and person-to-person communication to encourage people to adopt and sustain new health-related behaviour.

Person-to-person communication can take place almost anywhere – informally at the water-pump, among members of sports teams, during conversations with family and friends, or through presentations and discussions in classrooms, health clinics, community meetings, women's group meetings, adult literacy classes or work groups. Person-to-person communication provides opportunities to ask questions and resolve doubts, to discuss inhibiting factors and obstacles, and to develop solutions.

Effective learning involves a cycle of information, action and reflection. People learn best when they participate actively in identifying a problem, in developing and carrying out a solution, and in reviewing the results. The process of communicating *Facts for Life* messages should therefore allow the participants to play an active role.

● Begin a discussion of one of the problems that is important to the person or group. Start with what is already known and focus on major concerns. Avoid technical or scientific language.

● Encourage people to ask questions and air concerns. Guide the discussion to explore the causes of the problem and possible solutions.

● Remember to listen, which is just as important to communication as speaking. Listening helps to clarify why people are – or are not – taking the recommended action. Intermediate steps may be needed to address unforeseen problems that prevent people from acting on the health message.

● Show respect for other's opinions, knowledge and ability to change. People learn best in situations that build their confidence, and they take action when they feel understood and respected.

● Support the person or group in taking action to solve the problem.

● Provide assistance to monitor progress, assess the results of actions and consider any necessary changes or further action.

From information to action

The goal of *Facts for Life* is to reduce childhood illness and death. The publication recommends actions that may require fundamental changes in how people do certain things.

Behaviour is based on deeply held beliefs and cultural values, and changing behaviour requires confidence and courage. People may resist change because they lack understanding, motivation or the means to resolve the problem. The following chart shows how change takes place, evolving from lack of awareness of a problem to understanding the situation and taking action.

Obstacle	How to resolve it
Lack of awareness of the problem	▶ Use the mass media and/or person-to-person communication and advocacy to raise awareness of the problem.
Lack of understanding about the extent of the problem, its causes and its solution	▶ Provide information in an interesting way, using local examples.
Lack of understanding about how to resolve the problem	▶ Provide information, help people identify solutions and support development of new skills, if necessary. Facilitate discussion about what to do and how to do it. ▶ Discuss the strengths and weaknesses of the new behaviour and how it relates to, and builds on, existing knowledge and practices. ▶ Discuss what changes are possible now and what changes can be developed later in the process.
Need for support and encouragement	▶ Discuss the barriers and benefits of taking action at the individual, family and community level. Enlist influential local groups or individuals as partners in the process.
Need for motivation	▶ Facilitate changes and provide support. Encourage discussion of the changes.
Need to sustain the new behaviour	▶ Discuss what has resulted from taking action. If there have been unexpected or negative results, explore the causes and develop solutions. ▶ Follow up to monitor developments and maintain actions or consider new problems.

Thank you for your support in communicating the *Facts for Life* messages.

Facts for Life Lessons from Experience is a very useful publication that reviews numerous field experiences in using the two previous editions of *Facts for Life*. Complimentary copies are available in English, French and Spanish. Contact the nearest UNICEF office or UNICEF headquarters in New York to order. Use the order form on page 153.

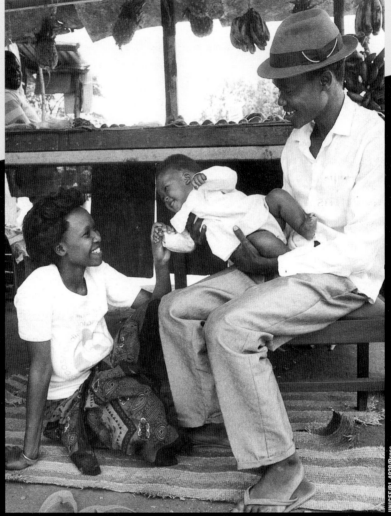

Why it is important to share and act on information about

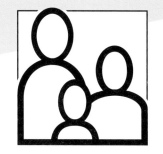

Timing Births

Too many births, births too close together, and births to adolescent girls or women over the age of 35 endanger women's lives and account for approximately one third of all infant deaths.

Family planning is one of the most powerful ways of improving the health of women and children. Over 100 million women in developing countries who are married or living with men report that their needs for contraception remain unmet. Access to family planning services for everyone, including adolescents, particularly in countries where marriage occurs early in life, together with universal access to education, would help prevent many maternal and child deaths and disabilities.

Key Messages:

What every family and community has a right to know about

Timing Births

1. Pregnancy before the age of 18 or after the age of 35 increases the health risks for the mother and her baby.

2. For the health of both mothers and children, there should be a space of at least two years between births.

3. The health risks of pregnancy and childbirth increase after four pregnancies.

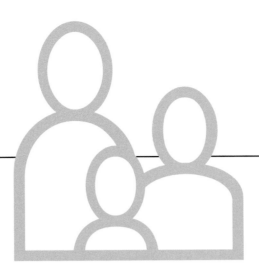

4. Family planning services provide people with the knowledge and the means to plan when to begin having children, how many to have and how far apart to have them, and when to stop. There are many safe and acceptable ways of avoiding pregnancy.

5. Family planning is the responsibility of both men and women; everyone needs to know about the health benefits.

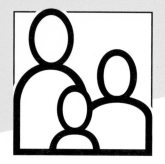

Timing Births

1. Pregnancy before the age of 18 or after the age of 35 increases the health risks for the mother and her baby.

Every year some 515,000 women die from problems linked to pregnancy and childbirth. For every woman who dies, approximately 30 more develop serious, disabling problems. Family planning could prevent many of these deaths and much of this disability.

Delaying a first pregnancy until a girl is at least 18 years of age will help ensure a safer pregnancy and delivery, and will reduce the risk of her baby being born underweight. This is especially important in countries where early marriage is the custom.

A girl is not physically ready to begin bearing children until she is about 18 years of age. Childbirth is more likely to be difficult and dangerous for an adolescent than for an adult. Babies born to very young mothers are much more likely to die in the first year of life. The younger the mother, the greater the risk to her and her baby.

Young women need special help to delay pregnancy. Young women and their families should be given information about the risks of early pregnancy and how to avoid them.

After the age of 35, the health risks of pregnancy and childbirth begin to increase again. If a woman is over the age of 35 and has had four or more pregnancies, another pregnancy is a serious risk to her own health and that of the foetus.

2. For the health of both mothers and children, there should be a space of at least two years between births.

The risk of death for young children increases by nearly 50 per cent if the space between births is less than two years.

One of the greatest threats to the health and growth of a child under the age of two is the birth of a new baby. Breastfeeding for the older child stops too soon, and the mother has less time to prepare the special foods a young child needs. She may not be able to give the older child the care and attention he or she needs, especially when the child is ill. As a result, children born less than two years apart usually do not develop as well, physically or mentally, as children born two years apart or more.

A woman's body needs two years to recover fully from pregnancy and childbirth. The risk to the mother's health is therefore greater if births come too close together. The mother needs time to get her health, nutritional status and energy back before she becomes pregnant again. Men need to be aware of the importance of a two-year space between births and the need to limit the number of pregnancies to help protect their family's health.

If a woman becomes pregnant before she is fully recovered from a previous pregnancy, there is a higher chance that her new baby will be born too early and weigh too little. Babies born underweight are less likely to grow well, more likely to become ill and four times more likely to die in the first year of life than babies of normal weight.

3. The health risks of pregnancy and childbirth increase after four pregnancies.

A woman's body can easily become exhausted by repeated pregnancies, childbirth, breastfeeding and caring for small children. After four pregnancies, especially if there has been less than two years between births, she faces an increased risk of serious health problems such as anaemia ('thin blood') and haemorrhage (heavy loss of blood).

A baby is at greater risk of dying if the mother has had four or more pregnancies.

4. Family planning services provide people with the knowledge and the means to plan when to begin having children, how many to have and how far apart to have them, and when to stop. There are many safe and acceptable ways of avoiding pregnancy.

Health clinics should offer advice to help people choose a family planning method that is acceptable, safe, convenient, effective and affordable.

Of the various contraceptive methods, only condoms protect against both pregnancy and sexually transmitted infections, including HIV/AIDS.

Exclusive breastfeeding can delay the return of the mother's fertility for approximately six months after childbirth. Exclusive breastfeeding provides a woman with 98 per cent protection from pregnancy, but only if her baby is under the age of six months, her menstrual periods have not returned, and the baby is breastfed on demand and exclusively – receiving no other foods or drinks.

5. Family planning is the responsibility of both men and women; everyone needs to know about the health benefits.

Men as well as women must take responsibility for preventing unplanned pregnancies. They should have access to information and advice from a health worker so that they are aware of the various methods of family planning that are available.

Information can also be obtained from a doctor, nurse, teacher, family planning clinic, and youth or women's organization.

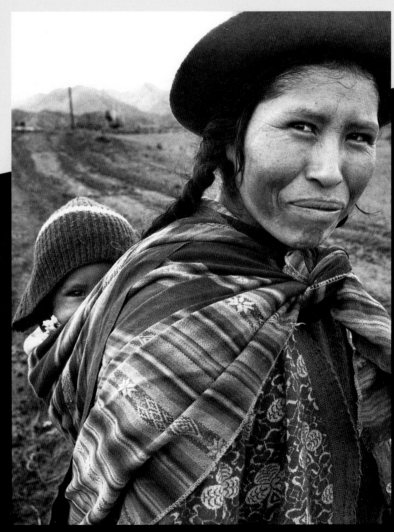

Why it is important to share and act on information about

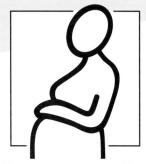

Safe Motherhood

Some 1,400 women die every day from problems related to pregnancy and childbirth. Tens of thousands more experience complications during pregnancy, many of which are life-threatening for the women and their children – or leave them with severe disabilities.

The dangers of childbearing can be greatly reduced if a woman is healthy and well nourished before becoming pregnant, if she has a health check-up by a trained health worker at least four times during every pregnancy, and if the birth is assisted by a skilled birth attendant such as a doctor, nurse or midwife. The woman should also be checked during the 12 hours after delivery and six weeks after giving birth.

Governments have a particular responsibility to make prenatal and postnatal services available, to train health workers to assist at childbirth, and to provide special care and referral services for women who have serious problems during pregnancy and childbirth.

Most governments have ratified an international agreement, the Convention on the Elimination of All Forms of Discrimination against Women, that includes a legally binding commitment to provide the services pregnant women need.

Key Messages:

**What every family and community
has a right to know about**

Safe Motherhood

1. It is important for all families to be able to recognize the warning signs of problems during pregnancy and childbirth and to have plans and resources for getting immediate skilled help if problems arise.

2. A skilled birth attendant, such as a doctor, nurse or trained midwife, should check the woman at least four times during every pregnancy and assist at every birth.

3. All pregnant women need particularly nutritious meals and more rest than usual throughout the pregnancy.

4. Smoking, alcohol, drugs, poisons and pollutants are especially harmful to pregnant women and young children.

  FACTS FOR LIFE

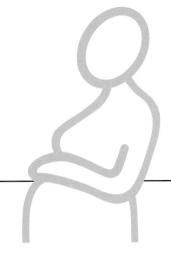

5. Physical abuse of women and children is a serious public health problem in many communities. Abuse during pregnancy is dangerous both to the woman and the foetus.

6. Girls who are educated, healthy and have a good diet during their childhood and teenage years will have fewer problems in pregnancy and childbirth.

7. Every woman has the right to health care, especially during pregnancy and childbirth. Health care providers should be technically competent and should treat women with respect.

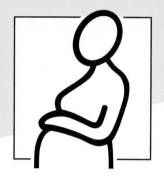

Safe Motherhood

1. It is important for all families to be able to recognize the warning signs of problems during pregnancy and childbirth and to have plans and resources for getting immediate skilled help if problems arise.

With any pregnancy there is a risk that something may go wrong. Most of these complications cannot be predicted. The first delivery is the most dangerous for both mother and child.

A pregnant woman needs to be checked at a clinic or health facility at least four times during every pregnancy. It is also important to seek the advice of a skilled birth attendant (such as a doctor, nurse or midwife) about where the baby should be born.

Because dangerous problems can arise without warning during pregnancy, childbirth or just after the birth, all families need to know the location of the nearest hospital or clinic and have plans and funds for quickly getting the woman there at any hour. If possible, the mother-to-be should move, temporarily, closer to a clinic or hospital so that she is within reach of medical help.

If a family knows that a birth is likely to be difficult or risky, the birth should take place in a hospital or maternity clinic. All births, especially first births, are safer in a maternity clinic or hospital.

All families need to know about special risk factors and be able to recognize the warning signs of possible problems.

Risk factors before pregnancy:

- an interval of less than two years since an earlier birth

- a girl is under 18 or a woman is over 35 years of age

- the woman already has four or more children

- the woman has had a previous premature birth or baby weighing less than 2 kilograms at birth

- the woman has had a previous difficult or Caesarean birth

- the woman has had a previous miscarriage or stillbirth

- the woman weighs less than 38 kilograms

- the woman has been through infibulation or genital cutting.

Warning signs during pregnancy:

- failure to gain weight (at least 6 kilograms should be gained during pregnancy)

- anaemia, paleness inside the eyelids (healthy eyelids are red or pink), very tired or easily out-of-breath

- unusual swelling of legs, arms or face

- the foetus moves very little or not at all.

Signs that mean get help immediately:

- spotting or bleeding from the vagina during pregnancy or profuse or persistent bleeding after delivery

- severe headaches or stomach-aches

- severe or persistent vomiting

SAFE MOTHERHOOD

- high fever

- the water breaks before due time for delivery

- convulsions

- severe pain

- prolonged labour.

2. A skilled birth attendant, such as a doctor, nurse or trained midwife, should check the woman at least four times during every pregnancy and assist at every birth.

Every pregnancy deserves attention, as there is always a risk of something going wrong. Many dangers can be avoided if the woman goes to a health centre or to a skilled birth attendant when she first suspects she is pregnant. She should then have at least four check-ups throughout each pregnancy and also be checked during the 12 hours following each delivery and six weeks after each birth.

If there is bleeding or abdominal pain during pregnancy or any of the warning signs listed above, a health worker or a skilled birth attendant should be consulted immediately.

Having a skilled birth attendant assist at the delivery in a health facility and check on the mother in the 12 hours after delivery reduces the likelihood of either the mother or the baby becoming ill or dying.

A skilled birth attendant (such as a doctor, nurse or trained midwife) will help ensure a safer pregnancy and healthy baby by:

- checking the progress of the pregnancy so that if problems arise the woman can be moved to a hospital for the birth

- checking for high blood pressure, which can be dangerous to both mother and child

- checking for anaemia and providing iron/folate supplements regularly

- prescribing an adequate dosage of vitamin A to protect the mother and her newborn baby against infection (in vitamin A deficient areas)

- checking any infections during pregnancy, especially urinary tract infections and sexually transmitted infections, and treating them with antibiotics

- giving the pregnant woman two injections to protect her and her newborn baby against tetanus

- encouraging all pregnant women to use only iodized salt in food preparation, to help protect them from goitre and their children from future mental and physical disabilities

- checking that the foetus is growing properly

- giving antimalarial tablets, if necessary

- preparing the mother for the experience of childbirth and giving advice on breastfeeding and caring for herself and her newborn

- advising the pregnant woman and her family on where the birth should take place and how to get help if problems arise during childbirth or immediately after delivery

- advising on how to avoid sexually transmitted infections

- providing voluntary and confidential HIV testing and counselling. All women have the right to voluntary and confidential HIV testing and counselling. Pregnant women or new mothers who are infected, or suspect that they may be infected, should consult a trained health worker for counselling on how to reduce the risk of infecting their infants and how to care for themselves.

SAFE MOTHERHOOD

During delivery, the skilled attendant knows:

- when labour has gone on for too long (over 12 hours) and when a move to a hospital is necessary

- when medical help is required and how to obtain it

- how to reduce the risk of infection (clean hands, clean instruments and a clean delivery area)

- what to do if the baby is in the wrong position

- what to do if the mother is losing too much blood

- when to cut the umbilical cord and how to care for it

- what to do if the baby does not begin breathing right away

- how to dry the baby and keep her or him warm after delivery

- how to guide the baby to breastfeed immediately after delivery

- how to deliver the afterbirth safely and care for the mother after the baby is born

- how to put recommended drops in the baby's eyes to prevent blindness.

After delivery, the skilled attendant should:

- check on the woman's health in the 12 hours after birth and six weeks after delivery

- advise women on how to prevent or postpone another birth

- advise women on how to avoid sexually transmitted infections such as HIV or how to reduce the risk of infecting their infants.

3. All pregnant women need particularly nutritious meals and more rest than usual throughout the pregnancy.

A pregnant woman needs the best foods available to the family: milk, fruit, vegetables, meat, fish, eggs, grains, peas and beans. All these foods are safe to eat during pregnancy.

Women will feel stronger and be healthier during pregnancy if they eat foods that are rich in iron, vitamin A and folic acid. These foods include meat, fish, eggs, green leafy vegetables, and orange or yellow fruits and vegetables. Health workers can provide pregnant women with iron tablets to prevent or treat anaemia and, in vitamin A deficient areas, an adequate dosage of vitamin A to help prevent infection. Pregnant women should not take more than 10,000 international units (IU) of vitamin A per day, or 25,000 IU per week.

Salt used should be iodized. Women who do not have enough iodine in their diet are more likely to have miscarriages and risk having an infant who is mentally or physically disabled. Goitre, a swelling at the front of the neck, is a clear sign that a woman is not getting enough iodine.

If anaemia, malaria or hookworms are suspected, the pregnant woman should consult a health worker.

SAFE MOTHERHOOD

4. Smoking, alcohol, drugs, poisons and pollutants are especially harmful to pregnant women and young children.

A pregnant woman can damage her own health and the health of the foetus by smoking or living in an environment where others smoke, by drinking alcohol or by using narcotic drugs. It is important not to take medicines during pregnancy unless they are absolutely necessary and prescribed by a trained health worker.

If a pregnant woman smokes, her child is likely to be born underweight and is also more likely to have coughs, colds, croup, pneumonia or other breathing problems.

To ensure the physical growth and mental development of the child, pregnant women and young children need to be protected from smoke from tobacco or cooking fires; from pesticides, herbicides and other poisons; and from pollutants such as lead, found in water transported by lead pipes, vehicle exhaust and some paints.

5. Physical abuse of women and children is a serious public health problem in many communities. Abuse during pregnancy is dangerous both to the woman and the foetus.

If a pregnant woman is abused, she and the foetus could be seriously harmed. Pregnant women who are physically abused may be unable to have any more children. Members of her family should be aware of these dangers and she should be protected from her abuser.

6. Girls who are educated, healthy and have a good diet during their childhood and teenage years will have fewer problems in pregnancy and childbirth.

Being able to read and write helps women protect their own and their family's health. Girls who have at least seven years of schooling are less likely to become pregnant during adolescence and are more likely to marry later than those with little or no education.

A nutritious diet during childhood and adolescence reduces problems in pregnancy and childbirth. A nutritious diet includes beans and other pulses, grains, green leafy vegetables, and red/yellow/orange vegetables and fruits. Whenever possible, milk or other dairy products, eggs, fish, chicken and meat should be included.

Genital cutting of girls or women can cause serious vaginal and urinary infections that can result in sterility and death. Female genital cutting can also cause dangerous complications during childbirth and mental health problems for girls and women.

7. Every woman has the right to health care, especially during pregnancy and childbirth. Health care providers should be technically competent and should treat women with respect.

If women have access to health care and professional advice during pregnancy, during delivery and after delivery, many dangers of pregnancy and childbirth can be avoided.

All women have the right to the services of a skilled birth attendant such as a doctor, nurse or midwife, and to emergency obstetric care if needed.

Quality health care enables women to make informed decisions about their health by offering information and counselling. It should be easy for women who need maternal care to reach the health facility, and cost should not prevent women from using these services. Health care providers should have the skills needed to provide quality care. They should be trained to treat all women with respect, to be sensitive to cultural norms and practices, and to respect women's right to confidentiality and privacy.

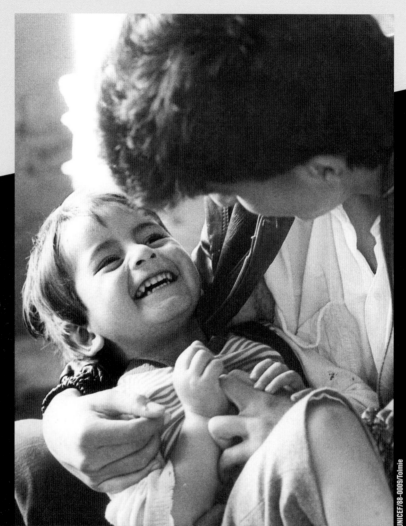

Why it is important to share and act on information about

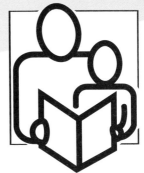

Child Development and Early Learning

The first eight years of childhood are critically important, particularly the first three years. They are the foundation of future health, growth and development. During this period, children learn more quickly than at any other time. Babies and young children develop more rapidly and learn more quickly when they receive love and affection, attention, encouragement and mental stimulation, as well as nutritious meals and good health care.

All children have the right to legal registration at birth, health care, good nutrition, education, and protection from harm, abuse and discrimination. It is the duty of parents and governments to ensure that these rights are respected, protected and fulfilled.

Key Messages:

What every family and community has a right to know about

Child Development and Early Learning

1. The care and attention a child receives in the first eight years of life, particularly during the first three years, are critically important and influence her or him for life.

2. Babies learn rapidly from the moment of birth. They grow and learn fastest when they receive affection, attention and stimulation in addition to good nutrition and proper health care.

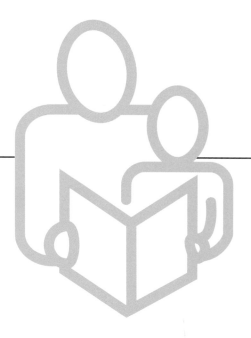

3. Encouraging children to play and explore helps them learn and develop socially, emotionally, physically and intellectually.

4. Children learn how to behave by imitating the behaviour of those closest to them.

5. All parents and caregivers should know the warning signs that show the child's growth and development are faltering.

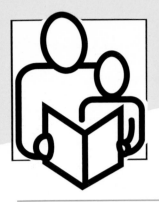

Child Development and Early Learning

1. The care and attention a child receives in the first eight years of life, particularly during the first three years, are critically important and influence her or him for life.

Care and affection during the first years help a child thrive. Holding, cuddling and talking to the child stimulate growth and promote emotional development. Being kept close to the mother and breastfed on demand also provide the infant with a sense of security. The baby needs to suckle for both nutrition and comfort.

Boys and girls have the same physical, mental, emotional and social needs. Both have the same capacity for learning. And both have the same need for affection, attention and approval.

Crying is a young child's way of communicating his or her needs. Responding promptly to the child's cry by holding and talking soothingly to her or him will help establish a sense of trust and security.

Children who are anaemic, malnourished or frequently sick may become fearful and upset more easily than healthy children and will lack the drive to play, explore and interact with others. These children need special attention and encouragement to eat.

Children's emotions are real and powerful. They may become frustrated if they are unable to do something or have something they want. Children are often frightened of strangers or the dark. Children whose reactions

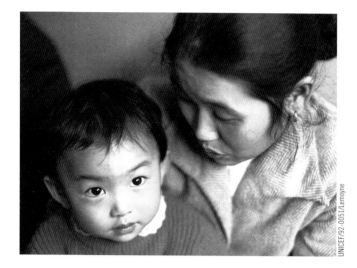

UNICEF/92-0051/Lemoyne

are laughed at, punished or ignored may grow up shy and unable to express emotions normally. If caregivers are patient and sympathetic when a child expresses strong emotions, the child is more likely to grow up happy, secure and well balanced.

Physical punishment or displays of violence can harm the child's development. Children who are punished in anger are more likely to become violent themselves. Clear explanations about what to do, firm rules about what not to do and praise for good behaviour are more effective ways of encouraging children to become full and productive members of the family and community.

Both parents, as well as other family members, need to be involved in caring for the children. The father's role is especially important. The father can help meet the child's needs for love, affection and stimulation and ensure the child receives a good quality education, good nutrition and health care. The father can help ensure that the environment is safe and free of violence. Fathers can also perform household tasks, particularly when the mother is pregnant or breastfeeding.

CHILD DEVELOPMENT & EARLY LEARNING

2. Babies learn rapidly from the moment of birth. They grow and learn fastest when they receive affection, attention and stimulation in addition to good nutrition and proper health care.

Skin-to-skin contact and breastfeeding within one hour after birth helps babies achieve better growth and development and establishes contact with their mother.

Touch, hearing, smell, sight and taste are learning tools the child uses to explore the surrounding world.

Children's minds develop rapidly when they are talked to, touched and cuddled, and when they see familiar faces, hear familiar voices and handle different objects. They learn quickly when they feel loved and secure from birth and when they frequently play and interact with family members. Children who feel secure usually do better in school and cope more easily with the difficulties of life.

Exclusive breastfeeding on demand for the first six months, timely introduction of safe and nutritious complementary foods at the age of six months, and continued breastfeeding for two years or beyond provide the child with nutrition and health benefits as well as affection and contact with the caregiver.

The most important way children develop and learn is through interaction with others. The more often parents and caregivers talk and respond to the child, the quicker he or she learns. Parents or caregivers should talk, read or sing to infants and young children. Even if children are not yet able to understand the words, these early 'conversations' develop their language and learning capacities.

Caregivers can help children learn and grow by giving them new and interesting things to look at, listen to, hold and play with.

Babies and small children should not be left alone for long periods of time. This delays their physical and mental development.

Girls need the same amount of food, attention, affection and care as do boys. All children need to be encouraged and praised when they learn to do and say new things.

When the child is not growing well, physically or mentally, parents need to seek advice from a health care worker.

Teaching children in their mother tongue first helps them develop their ability to think and express themselves. Children learn language quickly and easily through songs, family stories, rhymes and games.

A child who has completed immunization on time and has been given proper nutrition has an increased chance of survival and is more apt to interact, play and learn. This will reduce the family's expenditure on health care, the child's absence from school due to illness, and the parents' loss of income when they have to care for a sick child.

CHILD DEVELOPMENT
& EARLY LEARNING

3. Encouraging children to play and explore helps them learn and develop socially, emotionally, physically and intellectually.

Children play because it is fun, but play is also key to their learning and development. Playing builds children's knowledge and experience and helps develop their curiosity and confidence. Children learn by trying things, comparing results, asking questions and meeting challenges. Play develops the skills of language, thinking, planning, organizing and decision-making. Stimulation and play are especially important if the child has a disability.

Girls and boys need the same opportunities for play and for interaction with all family members. Play and interaction with the father help strengthen the bond between the father and the child.

Family members and other caregivers can help children learn by giving them simple tasks with clear instructions, providing objects to play with and suggesting new activities, but without dominating the child's play. Watch the child closely and follow her or his ideas.

Caregivers need to be patient when a very young child insists on trying to do something unaided. Children learn from trying until they succeed. As long as the child is protected from danger, struggling to do something new and difficult is a positive step in the child's development.

All children need a variety of simple materials to play with that are suitable for their stage of development. Water, sand, cardboard boxes, wooden building blocks, and pots and lids are just as good as toys bought from a shop.

Children are constantly changing and developing new abilities. Caregivers should notice these changes and follow the child's lead to help her or him develop more quickly.

4. Children learn how to behave by imitating the behaviour of those closest to them.

By watching and imitating others, young children learn how to interact socially. They learn what kinds of behaviour are and are not acceptable.

The examples set by adults and older children are the most powerful influences in shaping a child's behaviour and personality. Children learn by copying what others *do*, not what others *tell them to do*. If adults shout and behave violently, children will learn this type of behaviour. If adults treat others with kindness, respect and patience, children will follow their example.

Children like to pretend. This should be encouraged as it develops the child's imagination. It also helps the child understand and accept the ways other people behave.

5. All parents and caregivers should know the warning signs that show the child's growth and development are faltering.

Parents and caregivers need to know the major milestones that show the child is developing normally. They also need to know when to seek help and how to provide a caring and loving environment for a child with a physical or mental disability.

All children grow and develop in similar patterns, but each child develops at his or her own rate.

By observing young children to see how they respond to touch, sound and sight, parents can identify signs of possible developmental problems or disabilities. If a child is developing slowly, parents and caregivers can help by spending extra time with the child, playing and talking with the child, and massaging the child's body.

If the child does not respond to stimulation and attention, parents and caregivers need to seek help. Taking early action is very important in helping children with disabilities reach their full potential. Parents and caregivers need to encourage the greatest possible development of the child's abilities.

A girl or boy with a disability needs extra love and protection. Like all children, such a child needs to be registered at birth or soon afterwards, breastfed, immunized, given nutritious food and protected from abuse and violence. Children with disabilities should be encouraged to play and interact with other children.

A child who is unhappy or experiencing emotional difficulties may behave abnormally. Examples include suddenly becoming unfriendly, sad, lazy, unhelpful or naughty; crying often; becoming violent with other children; sitting alone instead of playing with friends; or suddenly having no interest in usual activities or school work and losing appetite and sleep.

- Parents should be encouraged to talk with and listen to the child and, if the problem persists, to seek help from a teacher or health worker.

- If a child has mental or emotional difficulties or has been abused, he or she should be given counselling to prevent further complications.

The following guide gives parents an idea of how children develop. There are differences in the growth and development of all children. Slow progress may be normal or may be due to inadequate nutrition, poor health, a lack of stimulation or a more serious problem. Parents may wish to discuss the child's progress with a trained health worker or a teacher.

How Children Develop

	By the age of ONE MONTH
A baby should be able to:	▶ turn her or his head towards a hand that is stroking the child's cheek or mouth ▶ bring both hands towards her or his mouth ▶ turn towards familiar voices and sounds ▶ suckle the breast and touch it with her or his hands.
Advice for parents and caregivers:	▶ make skin-to-skin contact and breastfeed within one hour of birth ▶ support the baby's head when you hold the baby upright ▶ massage and cuddle the baby often ▶ always handle the baby gently, even when you are tired or upset ▶ breastfeed frequently, at least every four hours ▶ talk, read and sing to the child as often as possible ▶ visit the health worker with the infant six weeks after birth.
Warning signs to watch for:	▶ poor suckling at the breast or refusing to suckle ▶ little movement of arms and legs ▶ little or no reaction to loud sounds or bright lights ▶ crying for long periods for no apparent reason ▶ vomiting and diarrhoea, which can lead to dehydration.

CHILD DEVELOPMENT & EARLY LEARNING

A baby should be able to:

▶ raise the head and chest when lying on her or his stomach

▶ reach for dangling objects

▶ grasp and shake objects

▶ roll both ways

▶ sit with support

▶ explore objects with hands and mouth

▶ begin to imitate sounds and facial expressions

▶ respond to her or his own name and to familiar faces.

Advice for parents and caregivers:

▶ lay the baby on a clean, flat, safe surface so she or he can move freely and reach for objects

▶ prop or hold the baby in a position so she or he can see what is happening nearby

▶ continue to breastfeed on demand day and night, and start adding other foods (two meals a day at 6-8 months, 3-4 meals a day at 8-12 months)

▶ talk, read or sing to the child as often as possible.

Warning signs to watch for:

▶ stiffness or difficulty moving limbs

▶ constant moving of the head (this might indicate an ear infection, which could lead to deafness if not treated)

▶ little or no response to sounds, familiar faces or the breast

▶ refusing the breast or other foods.

By the age of 12 MONTHS

A baby should be able to:

▶ sit without support

▶ crawl on hands and knees and pull up to stand

▶ take steps holding onto support

▶ try to imitate words and sounds and respond to simple requests

▶ enjoy playing and clapping

▶ repeat sounds and gestures for attention

▶ pick things up with thumb and one finger

▶ start holding objects such as a spoon and cup and attempt self-feeding.

Advice for parents and caregivers:

▶ point to objects and name them, talk and play with the child frequently

▶ use mealtimes to encourage interaction with all family members

▶ if the child is developing slowly or has a physical disability, focus on the child's abilities and give extra stimulation and interaction

▶ do not leave a child in one position for many hours

▶ make the area as safe as possible to prevent accidents

▶ continue to breastfeed and ensure that the child has enough food and a variety of family foods

▶ help the child experiment with spoon/cup feeding

▶ make sure that the child is fully immunized and receives all recommended doses of micronutrient supplements.

Warning signs to watch for:

▶ the child does not make sounds in response to others

▶ the child does not look at objects that move

▶ the child is listless and does not respond to the caregiver

▶ the child has no appetite or refuses food.

By the age of TWO YEARS

A child should be able to:

▶ walk, climb and run

▶ point to objects or pictures when they are named (e.g., nose, eyes)

▶ say several words together (from about 15 months)

▶ follow simple instructions

▶ scribble if given a pencil or crayon

▶ enjoy simple stories and songs

▶ imitate the behaviour of others

▶ begin to eat by herself or himself.

Advice for parents and caregivers:

▶ read, sing or play games with the child

▶ teach the child to avoid dangerous objects

▶ talk to the child normally – do not use baby talk

▶ continue to breastfeed and ensure the child has enough food and a variety of family foods

▶ encourage, but do not force, the child to eat

▶ provide simple rules and set reasonable expectations

▶ praise the child's achievements.

By the age of TWO YEARS *(continued)*

Warning signs to watch for:

▶ lack of response to others

▶ difficulty keeping balance while walking (see a trained health worker)

▶ injuries and unexplained changes in behaviour (especially if the child has been cared for by others)

▶ lack of appetite.

By the age of THREE YEARS

A child should be able to:

▶ walk, run, climb, kick and jump easily

▶ recognize and identify common objects and pictures by pointing

▶ make sentences of two or three words

▶ say her or his own name and age

▶ name colours

▶ understand numbers

▶ use make-believe objects in play

▶ feed herself or himself

▶ express affection.

Advice for parents and caregivers:

▶ read and look at books with the child and talk about the pictures

▶ tell the child stories and teach rhymes and songs

▶ give the child her or his own bowl or plate of food

▶ continue to encourage the child to eat, giving the child as much time as he or she needs

▶ help the child learn to dress, wash her or his hands and use the toilet.

CHILD DEVELOPMENT & EARLY LEARNING

Warning signs to watch for:

- loss of interest in playing
- frequent falling
- difficulty manipulating small objects
- failure to understand simple messages
- inability to speak using several words
- little or no interest in food.

By the age of FIVE YEARS

A child should be able to:

- move in a coordinated way
- speak in sentences and use many different words
- understand opposites (e.g., fat and thin, tall and short)
- play with other children
- dress without help
- answer simple questions
- count 5 to 10 objects
- wash her or his hands.

Advice for parents and caregivers:

- listen to the child
- interact frequently with the child
- if the child stutters, suggest she or he speak more slowly
- read and tell stories
- encourage the child to play and explore.

By the age of FIVE YEARS *(continued)*

*Warning signs
to watch for:*

▶ observe the roles children take in play. If the child
is fearful, angry or violent, these may be signs of
emotional problems or abuse.

CHILD DEVELOPMENT
& EARLY LEARNING

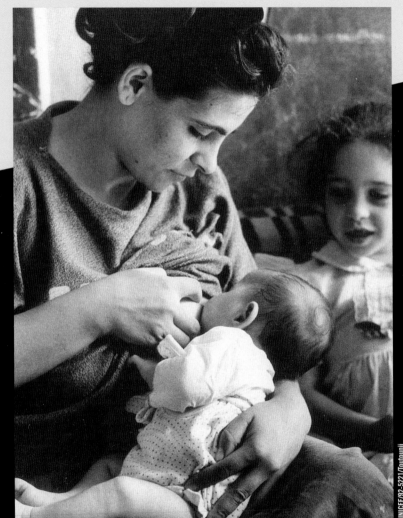

Why it is important to share and act on information about

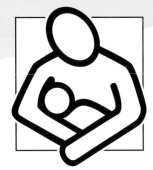

Breastfeeding

Babies who are breastfed have fewer illnesses and are better nourished than those who are fed other drinks and foods. If all babies were fed only breastmilk for the first six months of life, the lives of an estimated 1.5 million infants would be saved every year and the health and development of millions of others would be greatly improved.

Using breastmilk substitutes, such as infant formula or animal's milk, can be a threat to infants' health. This is particularly the case if parents cannot afford sufficient substitutes, which are quite expensive, or do not always have clean water with which to mix them.

Almost every mother can breastfeed successfully. Those who might lack the confidence to breastfeed need the encouragement and practical support of the baby's father and their family, friends and relatives. Health workers, women's organizations, the mass media and employers can also provide support.

Everyone should have access to information about the benefits of breastfeeding and it is the duty of every government to provide this information.

Key Messages:

What every family and community has a right to know about

Breastfeeding

1. Breastmilk *alone* is the only food and drink an infant needs for the first six months. No other food or drink, not even water, is usually needed during this period.

2. There is a risk that a woman infected with HIV can pass the disease on to her infant through breastfeeding. Women who are infected or suspect that they may be infected should consult a trained health worker for testing, counselling and advice on how to reduce the risk of infecting the child.

3. Newborn babies should be kept close to their mothers and begin breastfeeding within one hour of birth.

4. Frequent breastfeeding causes more milk to be produced. Almost every mother can breastfeed successfully.

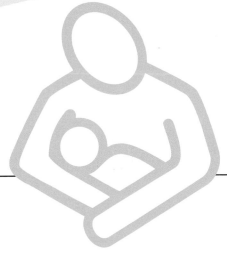

5. Breastfeeding helps protect babies and young children against dangerous illnesses. It also creates a special bond between mother and child.

6. Bottle-feeding can lead to illness and death. If a woman cannot breastfeed her infant, the baby should be fed breast-milk or a breastmilk substitute from an ordinary clean cup.

7. From the age of six months, babies need a variety of additional foods, but breastfeeding should continue through the child's second year and beyond.

8. A woman employed away from her home can continue to breastfeed her child if she breastfeeds as often as possible when she is with the infant.

9. Exclusive breastfeeding can give a woman more than 98 per cent protection against pregnancy for six months after giving birth – but only if her menstrual periods have not resumed, if her baby breastfeeds frequently day and night, and if the baby is not given any other food or drinks, or a pacifier or dummy.

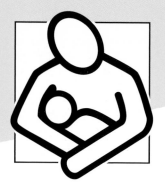

Breastfeeding

1. Breastmilk *alone* is the only food and drink an infant needs for the first six months. No other food or drink, not even water, is usually needed during this period.

Breastmilk is the best food a young child can have. Animal's milk, infant formula, powdered milk, teas, sugar drinks, water and cereal foods are inferior to breastmilk.

Breastmilk is easy for the baby to digest. It also promotes the best growth and development and protects against illness.

Even in hot, dry climates, breastmilk meets a young baby's need for fluids. Water or other drinks are not needed during the first six months. Giving a baby any food or drink other than breastmilk increases the risk of diarrhoea and other illnesses.

Breastmilk substitutes that are nutritionally adequate are expensive. For example, to feed one baby for a year requires 40 kilograms (about 80 tins) of infant formula. Health workers should inform all mothers who are considering the use of breastmilk substitutes about their cost.

If regular weighing shows that a breastfed baby under six months is not growing well:

● the child may need more frequent breastfeeding. At least 12 feeds during a 24-hour period may be necessary. The baby should suckle for at least 15 minutes.

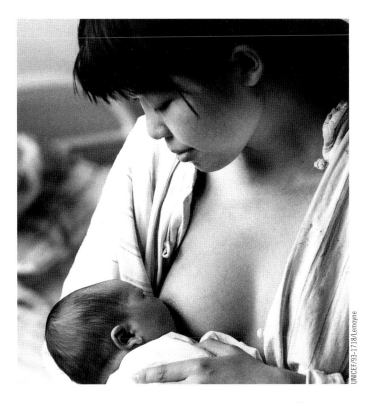

UNICEF/93-1718/Lemoyne

- the child may need help to take more of the breast into the mouth

- the child may be ill and should be taken to a trained health worker

- water or other fluids may be reducing the intake of breastmilk. The mother should not give other fluids and should breastfeed only.

Any infant older than six months of age needs other foods and drinks. Breastfeeding should also continue until the child is two years or older.

BREASTFEEDING

2. **There is a risk that a woman infected with HIV can pass the disease on to her infant through breastfeeding. Women who are infected or suspect that they may be infected should consult a trained health worker for testing, counselling and advice on how to reduce the risk of infecting the child.**

It is important for everyone to know how to avoid HIV infection. Pregnant women and new mothers should be aware that if they are infected with HIV they may infect their infant during pregnancy or childbirth or through breastfeeding.

The best way to avoid the risk of transmitting the infection is to avoid becoming infected. The risk of sexual transmission of HIV can be reduced if people don't have sex, if uninfected partners have sex only with each other, or if people have safer sex – sex without penetration or while using a condom.

Pregnant women or new mothers who are infected or suspect that they are infected should consult a qualified health worker to seek testing and counselling.

3. **Newborn babies should be kept close to their mothers and begin breastfeeding within one hour of birth.**

A newborn baby needs to remain in skin-to-skin contact with the mother as much as possible. It is best for the mother and baby to stay together in the same room or bed. The baby should be allowed to breastfeed as often as he or she wants.

Having the baby start to breastfeed soon after birth stimulates the production of the mother's breastmilk. It also helps the mother's uterus contract, which reduces the risk of heavy bleeding or infection.

Colostrum, the thick yellowish milk the mother produces in the first few days after birth, is the perfect food for newborn babies. It is very nutritious and helps protect the baby against infections. Sometimes mothers are advised not to feed colostrum to their babies. *This advice is incorrect.*

The baby needs no other food or drink while waiting for the mother's milk supply to increase.

If a mother gives birth in a hospital or clinic, she has a right to expect that her baby will be kept near her in the same room, 24 hours a day, and that no formula or water will be given to her baby if she is breastfeeding.

4. Frequent breastfeeding causes more milk to be produced. Almost every mother can breastfeed successfully.

Many new mothers need encouragement and help to begin breastfeeding. Another woman who has successfully breastfed or a family member, friend or member of a women's breastfeeding support group can help a mother overcome uncertainties and prevent difficulties.

How the mother holds her baby and how the baby takes the breast in the mouth are very important. Holding the baby in a good position makes it easier for the baby to take the breast well into the mouth and suckle.

Signs that the baby is in a good position for breastfeeding are:

- the baby's whole body is turned towards the mother
- the baby is close to the mother
- the baby is relaxed and happy.

Holding the baby in a poor suckling position can cause such difficulties as:

- sore and cracked nipples
- not enough milk
- refusal to feed.

FACTS FOR LIFE 45

Signs that the baby is feeding well:

- the baby's mouth is wide open

- the baby's chin is touching the mother's breast

- more of the dark skin around the mother's nipple can be seen above the baby's mouth than below it

- the baby takes long, deep sucks

- the mother does not feel any pain in the nipple.

Almost every mother can produce enough milk when:

- she breastfeeds exclusively

- the baby is in a good position and has the breast well in the mouth

- the baby feeds as often and for as long as he or she wants, including during the night.

From birth, the baby should breastfeed whenever he or she wants to. If a newborn sleeps more than three hours after breastfeeding, he or she may be gently awakened and offered the breast.

Crying is not a sign that the baby needs other foods or drinks. It normally means that the baby needs to be held and cuddled more. Some babies need to suckle the breast for comfort. More suckling will produce more breastmilk.

Mothers who fear that they do not have enough breastmilk often give their babies other food or drink in the first few months of life. But this causes the baby to suckle less often, so less breastmilk is produced. The mother will produce more milk if she does not give the child other food or drink and breastfeeds often.

 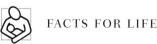

Pacifiers, dummies or bottles should not be given to breastfed babies because the sucking action for these is very different from suckling at the breast. Using pacifiers or bottles could cause the mother to produce less breast-milk and the baby to reduce or stop breastfeeding.

Mothers need to be reassured that they can feed their young babies properly with breastmilk alone. They need encouragement and support from the child's father, their families, neighbours, friends, health workers, employers and women's organizations.

Breastfeeding can provide an opportunity for a mother to rest. Fathers and other family members can help by encouraging the mother to rest quietly while she breast-feeds the baby. They can also make sure the mother has enough food and help with household tasks.

5. Breastfeeding helps protect babies and young children against dangerous illnesses. It also creates a special bond between mother and child.

Breastmilk is the baby's 'first immunization'. It helps to protect against diarrhoea, ear and chest infections and other health problems. The protection is greatest when breastmilk alone is given for the first six months and breastfeeding continues well into the second year and beyond. No other drinks or foods can provide this protection.

Breastfed babies usually get more attention and stimu-lation than those who are left to feed themselves with bottles. Attention helps infants grow and develop and helps them feel more secure.

BREASTFEEDING

6. Bottle-feeding can lead to illness and death. If a woman cannot breastfeed her infant, the baby should be fed breastmilk or a breastmilk substitute from an ordinary clean cup.

Unclean bottles and teats can cause illnesses such as diarrhoea and ear infections. Diarrhoea can be deadly for babies. Illness is less likely if the bottles and teats are sterilized in boiling water before each feed, but bottle-fed babies are still far more susceptible to diarrhoea and other common infections than breastfed babies.

The best food for a baby who cannot be breastfed is milk expressed from the mother's breast or from another healthy mother. The breastmilk should be given from a clean, open cup. Even newborn babies can be fed with an open cup, which can be easily cleaned.

The best food for any baby whose own mother's milk is not available is the breastmilk of another healthy mother.

If breastmilk is not available, a nutritionally adequate breastmilk substitute should be fed to the baby by cup. Infants who are fed breastmilk substitutes are at greater risk of death and disease than breastfed infants.

Feeding the baby breastmilk substitutes can cause poor growth or illness if too much or too little water is added or the water is not clean. It is important to boil and then cool the water and carefully follow the directions for mixing breastmilk substitutes.

Animal's milk and infant formula go bad if left at room temperature for a few hours. Breastmilk can be stored for up to eight hours at room temperature without going bad. Keep it in a clean, covered container.

7. From the age of six months, babies need a variety of additional foods, but breastfeeding should continue through the child's second year and beyond.

Although children need additional foods after they are six months old, breastmilk is still an important source of energy, protein and other nutrients such as vitamin A and iron. Breastmilk helps protect against disease for as long as the child breastfeeds. From the age of six months to one year, breastfeeding should be offered before other foods, to be sure the infant takes plenty of breastmilk every day. The child's diet should include peeled, cooked and mashed vegetables, grains, pulses and fruit, some oil, as well as fish, eggs, chicken, meat or dairy products to provide vitamins and minerals. In the second year, breastfeeding should be offered after meals and at other times. A mother can continue to breastfeed her child for as long as she and the child wish.

The general guidelines for complementary feeding are:

From 6 to 12 months: Breastfeed frequently and give other foods three to five times a day.

From 12 to 24 months: Breastfeed frequently and give family foods five times a day.

From 24 months onward: Continue breastfeeding if both mother and child wish and give family foods five times a day.

Babies fall ill frequently as they begin to crawl, walk, play, drink and eat foods other than breastmilk. A sick child needs plenty of breastmilk. Breastmilk is a nutritious, easily digestible food when a child loses appetite for other foods.

Breastfeeding can comfort a child who is upset.

BREASTFEEDING

8. A woman employed away from her home can continue to breastfeed her child if she breastfeeds as often as possible when she is with the infant.

If a mother cannot be with her baby during working hours, she should breastfeed often when they are together. Frequent breastfeeding will ensure her milk supply.

If a woman cannot breastfeed at her workplace, she should express her milk two or three times during the working day and save it in a clean container. Breastmilk can be stored for up to eight hours at room temperature without going bad. The expressed milk can be given to the child from a clean cup.

The mother should not give breastmilk substitutes.

Families and communities can encourage employers to provide paid maternity leave, crèches, and the time and a suitable place for women to breastfeed or express their milk.

9. Exclusive breastfeeding can give a woman more than 98 per cent protection against pregnancy for six months after giving birth — but only if her menstrual periods have not resumed, if her baby breastfeeds frequently day and night, and if the baby is not given any other food or drinks, or a pacifier or dummy.

The more often a baby breastfeeds, the longer it will take for the mother's menstrual periods to resume. If a mother breastfeeds less than eight times in 24 hours or gives other foods or drinks, or a pacifier or a dummy, the baby may breastfeed less often, causing the mother's periods to resume sooner.

It is possible for a mother to become pregnant before her periods return. This becomes increasingly likely six months after the birth.

A woman who wants to delay another pregnancy should choose another method of family planning if *any* of the following apply:

- her periods have resumed

- her baby is taking other food or drinks, or uses a pacifier or dummy

- her baby has reached the age of six months.

It is best for the health of the mother and her children if she avoids becoming pregnant again until her youngest child is more than two years of age. All new parents should be given family planning advice by a health worker or trained birth attendant.

Most methods of postponing pregnancy have no effect on the quality of the breastmilk. However, some contraceptive pills contain oestrogen, which can reduce the quantity of breastmilk. Trained health workers can provide advice about the best kind of contraception for a breastfeeding mother.

BREASTFEEDING

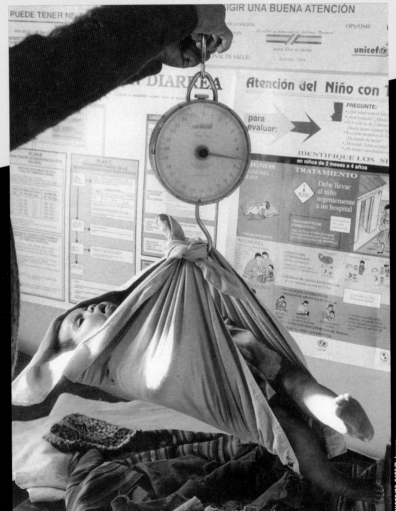

Why it is important to share and act on information about

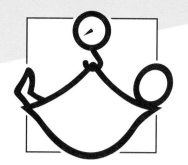

Nutrition and Growth

More than half of all child deaths are associated with malnutrition, which weakens the body's resistance to illness. Poor diet, frequent illness, and inadequate or inattentive care of young children can lead to malnutrition.

If a woman is malnourished during pregnancy, or if her child is malnourished during the first two years of life, the child's physical and mental growth and development may be slowed. This cannot be made up when the child is older – it will affect the child for the rest of his or her life.

Children have the right to a caring, protective environment and to nutritious food and basic health care to protect them from illness and promote growth and development.

Key
Messages:

**What every family and community
has a right to know about**

Nutrition
and Growth

1. A young child should grow well and gain weight rapidly. From birth to age two, children should be weighed every month. If a child has not gained weight for about two months, something is wrong.

2. Breastmilk alone is the only food and drink an infant needs until the age of six months. After six months, the child needs a variety of other foods in addition to breastmilk.

3. From the age of six months to two years, children need to be fed five times a day, in addition to sustained breastfeeding.

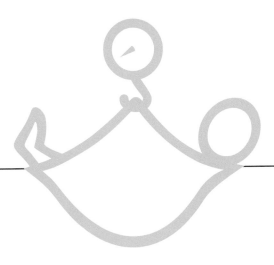

4. Children need vitamin A to resist illness and prevent visual impairments. Vitamin A can be found in many fruits and vegetables, oils, eggs, dairy products, fortified foods, breastmilk, or vitamin A supplements.

5. Children need iron-rich foods to protect their physical and mental abilities. The best sources of iron are liver, lean meats, fish, eggs and iron-fortified foods or iron supplements.

6. Iodized salt is essential to prevent learning disabilities and delayed development in children.

7. During an illness, children need to continue to eat regularly. After an illness, children need at least one extra meal every day for at least a week.

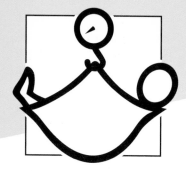

Nutrition
and Growth

1. A young child should grow well and gain weight rapidly. From birth to age two, children should be weighed every month. If a child has not gained weight for about two months, something is wrong.

Regular weight gain is the most important sign that a child is growing and developing well. The child should be weighed during every visit to a health centre.

A child who is given only breastmilk for about the first six months usually grows well during this time. Breastfeeding helps protect babies from common illnesses and ensures good physical and mental growth and development. Infants who are not breastfed may not learn as easily as breastfed infants.

If a child does not gain weight for two months, he or she may need larger servings or more nutritious food, may be sick or may need more attention and care. Parents and health workers need to act quickly to discover the cause of the problem.

Each young child should have a growth chart. The child's weight should be marked with a dot on the growth chart each time he or she is weighed, and the dots should be connected after each weighing. This will produce a line that shows how well the child is growing. If the line goes up, the child is doing well. A line that stays flat or goes down indicates cause for concern.

If a child is not regularly gaining weight or growing well, there are some important questions to ask:

 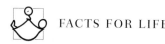

- **Is the child eating often enough?** A child needs to eat three to five times a day. A child with disabilities may require extra help and time for feeding.

- **Is the child receiving enough food?** If the child finishes his or her food and wants more, the child needs to be offered more.

- **Do the child's meals have too little 'growth' or 'energy' foods?** Foods that help the child grow are meat, fish, eggs, beans, nuts, grains and pulses. A small amount of oil will add energy. Red palm oil or other vitamin-enriched edible oils are good sources of energy.

- **Is the child refusing to eat?** If the child does not seem to like the taste of a particular food, other foods should be offered. New foods should be introduced gradually.

- **Is the child sick?** A sick child needs encouragement to eat small, frequent meals. After an illness, the child needs an extra meal every day for a week. Young children need extra breastmilk for at least a week. If the child is frequently ill, he or she should be checked by a trained health worker.

- **Is the child getting enough foods with vitamin A to prevent illness?** Breastmilk is rich in vitamin A. Other foods with vitamin A are liver, eggs, dairy products, red palm oil, yellow and orange fruits and vegetables, and many green leafy vegetables. If these foods are not available in adequate amounts, as is the case in many developing countries, a child needs a vitamin A capsule twice a year.

- **Is the child being given breastmilk substitutes by bottle?** If the child is younger than six months, exclusive breastfeeding is best. From 6 to 24 months breastmilk continues to be the best milk as it is an important source of many nutrients. If other milk is

FACTS FOR LIFE 57

given, it should be fed from a clean, open cup, rather than from a bottle.

- *Are food and water kept clean?* If not, the child will often be ill. Raw food should be washed or cooked. Cooked food should be eaten without delay. Leftover food should be thoroughly reheated.

  Water should come from a safe source and be kept clean. Clean drinking water can be obtained from a regularly maintained, controlled and chlorinated piped supply. Clean water can also be obtained from a tubewell, handpump, protected spring or well. If water is drawn from ponds, streams, springs, wells or tanks, it can be made safer by boiling.

- *Are faeces being put in a latrine or toilet or buried?* If not, the child may frequently get worms and other sicknesses. A child with worms needs deworming medicine from a health worker.

- *Is the young child left alone much of the time or in the care of an older child?* If so, the young child may need more attention from adults and more stimulation, especially during meals.

2. Breastmilk alone is the only food and drink an infant needs until the age of six months. After six months, the child needs a variety of other foods in addition to breastmilk.

In the early months, when the baby is most at risk, exclusive breastfeeding helps to protect against diarrhoea and other common infections. By about six months, a child needs other types of foods and drinks. Breastfeeding should continue into the second year.

If an infant under six months of age is not gaining weight, he or she may need to breastfeed more frequently.

- A breastfed infant under six months needs no other fluids, not even water.

- A breastfed infant who is not gaining weight may be ill, or may not be getting enough breastmilk. A health worker can check the infant's health and counsel the mother on how to increase the infant's intake of breastmilk.

Starting at about six months of age, infants need other foods, called complementary foods, in addition to breastmilk. The child's diet should include peeled, cooked and mashed vegetables, grains, pulses and fruit, some oil, as well as fish, eggs, chicken, meat or dairy products to provide vitamins and minerals. The greater the variety of foods, the better.

- Babies aged 6 to 12 months should be breastfed frequently and before being given other foods.

- After six months of age, the risk of infection increases as the child begins to eat other foods and starts to crawl. Both the child's hands and the child's food should be kept clean.

- Children aged 12 to 24 months should continue to breastfeed after meals and whenever they wish.

3. From the age of six months to two years, children need to be fed five times a day, in addition to sustained breastfeeding.

Poor nutrition in the first two years can slow a child's physical and mental development for the rest of her or his life.

In order to grow and stay healthy, young children need a variety of nutritious foods such as meat, fish, pulses, grains, eggs, fruits and vegetables, as well as breastmilk.

A child's stomach is smaller than an adult's, so a child cannot eat as much at one meal. But children's energy and body-building needs are great. So it is important that children eat frequently to provide for all their needs.

NUTRITION AND GROWTH

- Foods such as mashed vegetables, a little chopped meat, eggs or fish should be added to the child's food as often as possible. A small amount of oil may be added, preferably red palm oil or another vitamin-enriched oil.

If meals are served in a common dish, younger children may not get enough food. Young children should have their own plate or bowl of food to ensure they can eat what they need and so the parent or caregiver can see how much they have eaten.

Young children may need encouragement to eat and may need help in handling food or utensils. A child with a disability may need extra help eating and drinking.

4. Children need vitamin A to resist illness and prevent visual impairments. Vitamin A can be found in many fruits and vegetables, oils, eggs, dairy products, fortified foods, breastmilk, or vitamin A supplements.

Until children are six months of age, breastmilk provides them with all the vitamin A they need, provided the mother has enough vitamin A from her diet or supplements. Children six months and older need to get vitamin A from other foods or supplements.

Vitamin A can be found in liver, eggs, dairy products, fatty fish liver oil, ripe mangoes and papayas, yellow sweet potatoes, dark green leafy vegetables and carrots.

When children do not have enough vitamin A, they are at risk of night blindness. If the child has difficulty seeing in the early evening and at night, more vitamin A is probably needed. The child should be taken to a health worker for a vitamin A capsule.

In some countries, vitamin A has been added to oil and other foods. Vitamin A is also available in capsule or liquid form. In many countries vitamin A capsules are distributed once or twice a year to all children between six months and five years of age.

Diarrhoea and measles deplete vitamin A from the child's body. Vitamin A can be replaced by more frequent breastfeeding and, for children older than six months, by feeding the child more fruits and vegetables, eggs, liver and dairy products. Children with diarrhoea that lasts for more than 14 days and children with measles should be given a vitamin A capsule obtained from a health worker.

5. Children need iron-rich foods to protect their physical and mental abilities. The best sources of iron are liver, lean meats, fish, eggs and iron-fortified foods or iron supplements.

Anaemia – a lack of iron – can impair physical and mental development. Symptoms of anaemia include paleness of the tongue, the palms of the hands and the inside of the lips, tiredness and breathlessness. Anaemia is the most common nutritional disorder in the world.

● Even mild anaemia in infants and young children can impair intellectual development.

● Anaemia in children under two years of age may cause problems with coordination and balance, and the child may appear withdrawn and hesitant. This can limit the child's ability to interact and may hinder intellectual development.

Anaemia in pregnancy increases the severity of haemorrhage and the risk of infection during birth and is therefore a significant cause of maternal mortality. Infants born to anaemic mothers often suffer from low birthweight and anaemia. Iron supplements for pregnant women protect both women and their babies.

Iron is found in liver, lean meats, eggs and pulses. Fortifying foods with iron also prevents anaemia.

NUTRITION AND GROWTH

Malaria and hookworm can cause or worsen anaemia.

- Malaria can be prevented by sleeping under a mosquito net that has been treated with a recommended insecticide.

- Children living in areas where worms are highly endemic should be treated two to three times a year with a recommended antihelminthic medication. Good hygiene practices prevent worms. Children should not play near the latrine, should wash their hands often and should wear shoes to prevent worm infestations.

6. Iodized salt is essential to prevent learning disabilities and delayed development in children.

Small amounts of iodine are essential for children's growth and development. If a child does not get enough iodine, or if his or her mother is iodine-deficient during pregnancy, the child is likely to be born with a mental, hearing or speech disability, or may have delayed physical or mental development.

Goitre, a swelling of the neck, is one sign of a shortage of iodine in the diet. A pregnant woman with goitre is at high risk of miscarriage, stillbirth or of giving birth to a child with brain damage.

Using iodized salt instead of ordinary salt provides pregnant women and children with as much iodine as they need. If iodized salt is not available, women and children should receive iodine supplements from a health worker.

7. **During an illness, children need to continue to eat regularly. After an illness, children need at least one extra meal every day for at least a week.**

When children are sick, especially when they have diarrhoea or measles, their appetite decreases and their body uses the food they eat less effectively. If this happens several times a year, the child's growth will slow or stop.

It is essential to encourage a sick child to eat. This can be difficult, as children who are ill may have no appetite. It is important to keep offering foods the child likes, a little at a time and as often as possible. Extra breastfeeding is especially important.

It is essential to encourage a sick child to drink as often as possible. Dehydration is a serious problem for children with diarrhoea. Drinking plenty of liquids will help prevent dehydration.

If illness and poor appetite persist for more than a few days, the child needs to be taken to a health worker. The child is not fully recovered from an illness until he or she weighs about as much as when the illness began.

NUTRITION AND GROWTH

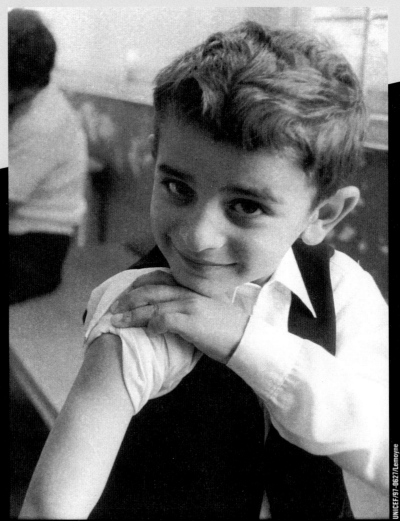

Why it is important to share and act on information about

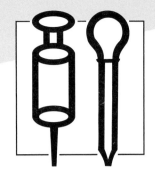

Immunization

Each year, 1.7 million children die from diseases that could have been prevented with readily available vaccines. Children who are immunized are protected from these dangerous diseases, which often lead to disability or death. All children have the right to this protection.

Every girl and boy needs to be immunized. And pregnant women need to be immunized to protect themselves and their infants from tetanus.

It is essential that all parents know why, when, where and how many times the child should be immunized. Parents also need to know that it is safe to immunize the child even if the child has an illness or a disability or is suffering from malnutrition.

Key Messages:

What every family and community has a right to know about

Immunization

1. Immunization is urgent. Every child needs a series of immunizations during the first year of life.

2. Immunization protects against several dangerous diseases. A child who is not immunized is more likely to suffer illness, become permanently disabled or become undernourished and die.

3. It is safe to immunize a child who has a minor illness, a disability or who is malnourished.

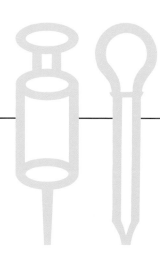

4. All pregnant women need to be protected against tetanus. Even if the woman was immunized earlier, she may need additional tetanus toxoid vaccinations. Check with a health worker for advice and tetanus toxoid immunization.

5. A new or sterile needle and syringe must be used for every person being immunized. People should insist on this.

6. Disease can spread quickly when people are crowded together. All children living in congested conditions, particularly in refugee or disaster situations, should be immunized immediately, especially against measles.

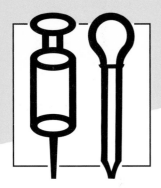

Immunization

1. Immunization is urgent. Every child needs a series of immunizations during the first year of life.

Children must be immunized early in life. Half of all deaths from whooping cough, a third of all cases of polio and a quarter of all deaths from measles occur in children under one year old.

It is essential that infants complete the *full* number of immunizations – otherwise the vaccines may not work.

To protect the child during the first year of life, the immunizations in the chart on page 69 are necessary. The immunizations are most effective if they are given at the ages specified, or as close to those ages as possible.

If for any reason a child has not had the full series of immunizations in the first year of life, it is extremely important to have the child fully immunized as soon as possible or during special National Immunization Days.

In some countries, additional vaccine doses, called 'booster shots', are offered after the first year of life. These shots make the vaccine protection even more effective.

Immunization schedule for infants*

Age	Immunizations to be given
At birth	BCG**, polio and, in some countries, hepatitis B
6 weeks	DPT**, polio and, in some countries, hepatitis B and Hib
10 weeks	DPT, polio and, in some countries, hepatitis B and Hib
14 weeks	DPT, polio and, in some countries, hepatitis B and Hib
9 months	Measles (12-15 months in industrialized countries) and, in some countries, yellow fever, mumps and rubella

*National immunization schedules may differ slightly from country to country.

**BCG offers partial protection against some forms of tuberculosis and leprosy; DPT protects against diphtheria, pertussis (whooping cough) and tetanus.

2. Immunization protects against several dangerous diseases. A child who is not immunized is more likely to suffer illness, become permanently disabled or become undernourished and die.

Immunization protects children against some of the most dangerous diseases of childhood. All children, including those who are disabled, need to be vaccinated. A child is immunized by vaccines, which are injected or given by mouth. The vaccines work by building up the child's defences against disease. Immunization only works if given *before* the disease strikes.

A child who is not immunized is very likely to get measles, whooping cough and other diseases that can kill. Children who survive these diseases are weakened and may not grow well or may be permanently disabled. They may die later from malnutrition and other illnesses.

All children need to be immunized against measles, which is a major cause of malnutrition, poor mental development, and hearing and visual impairments. The signs that a child has measles are a fever and rash that have lasted for three days or more, together with a cough, a runny nose or red eyes. Measles can cause death.

All children, everywhere, need to be immunized against polio. The signs of polio are a floppy limb or the inability to move. For every 200 children who are infected, one will be disabled for life.

Tetanus bacteria or spores, which grow in dirty cuts, can be deadly without a tetanus immunization.

- Immunizing a woman with at least two doses of tetanus toxoid before or during pregnancy protects not only the woman but also her newborn for the first weeks of the baby's life.

- At six weeks of age, the baby needs the first dose of DPT to extend the protection against tetanus.

In countries where hepatitis B is a problem, up to 10 out of every 100 children will harbour the infection for life if they are not immunized. Children who are infected with hepatitis B are likely to develop liver cancer when they are older.

In some countries, epidemics of yellow fever put many young children's lives at risk. Vaccination can prevent the disease.

In many countries, pneumonia caused by the *Haemophilus influenzae* type B (Hib) germ kills many young children. The Hib germ can also cause childhood meningitis. This germ is one of the most dangerous for children, particularly for those under five. Hib immunization can prevent these deaths.

Breastmilk and colostrum, the thick yellow milk produced during the first few days after birth, provide protection against pneumonia, diarrhoea and other diseases. Protection lasts for as long as the child is breastfed.

Vitamin A helps children fight infections and prevents blindness. Vitamin A is found in breastmilk, liver, fish, dairy products, some orange and yellow fruits and vegetables, and some green leafy vegetables. In areas of vitamin A deficiency, children aged six months and older should be given vitamin A capsules or liquid when they are immunized or during National Immunization Days. Vitamin A is also an important part of measles treatment.

3. It is safe to immunize a child who has a minor illness, a disability or who is malnourished.

One of the main reasons why parents do not bring a child for immunization is that the child has a fever, a cough, a cold, diarrhoea or some other illness on the day the child is to be immunized. However, it is safe to immunize a child who has a minor illness.

Sometimes a health worker advises against immunizing a child who has a disability or is malnourished. *This is wrong advice.* It is safe to immunize children who are disabled or malnourished.

After an injection, the child may cry or develop a fever, a minor rash or a small sore. This is normal. Breastfeed frequently or give the child plenty of liquids and foods. If the child has a high fever, the child should be taken to a health centre.

Because measles can be extremely dangerous for malnourished children, they should be immunized against measles, especially if the malnutrition is severe.

4. **All pregnant women need to be protected against tetanus. Even if the woman was immunized earlier, she may need additional tetanus toxoid vaccinations. Check with a health worker for advice and tetanus toxoid immunization.**

In many parts of the world, mothers give birth in unhygienic conditions. This puts both mother and child at risk of getting tetanus, a major killer of newborn infants.

If a pregnant woman is not immunized against tetanus and tetanus bacteria or spores enter her body, her life will also be at risk.

Tetanus bacteria or spores grow in dirty cuts. These germs can grow if the umbilical cord is cut with an unclean knife or if anything unclean touches the end of the cord. Any tool used to cut the cord should first be cleaned and then boiled or heated over a flame and allowed to cool. For the first week after birth, the baby's umbilical cord must be kept clean.

All pregnant women should check to make sure they have been immunized against tetanus. This protects both mothers and their newborn babies.

It is safe for a pregnant woman to be immunized against tetanus. She should be immunized according to this schedule:

First dose: As soon as she knows she is pregnant.

Second dose: One month after the first dose, and no later than two weeks before her due date.

Third dose: Six to 12 months after the second dose, or during the next pregnancy.

Fourth dose: One year after the third dose, or during a subsequent pregnancy.

Fifth dose: One year after the fourth dose, or during a subsequent pregnancy.

If a girl or a woman has been vaccinated with five properly spaced doses, she is protected for her lifetime. Her children are also protected for the first few weeks of life.

5. **A new or sterile needle and syringe must be used for every person being immunized. People should insist on this.**

Needles and equipment that are not properly sterilized can cause life-threatening disease. Sharing of syringes and needles, even among family members, can spread life-threatening disease. Only new or sterile needles and syringes should be used.

6. **Disease can spread quickly when people are crowded together. All children living in congested conditions, particularly in refugee or disaster situations, should be immunized immediately, especially against measles.**

Emergencies and situations that make people flee their homes often lead to the spread of communicable diseases. Therefore, all displaced children under 12 years of age should be immediately immunized, especially for measles, at the first point of contact or settlement.

All immunizations in emergency settings should be given with auto-disable syringes – syringes that can be used only once.

Measles is even more serious when children are malnourished or living in conditions of poor sanitation.

- As diseases like measles spread very quickly, a child with measles needs to be isolated from other children and examined by a trained health worker.

- Measles frequently causes severe diarrhoea. Immunizing children against measles prevents diarrhoea.

If routine child immunization has been disrupted, consult a health worker to complete the immunizations according to national guidelines.

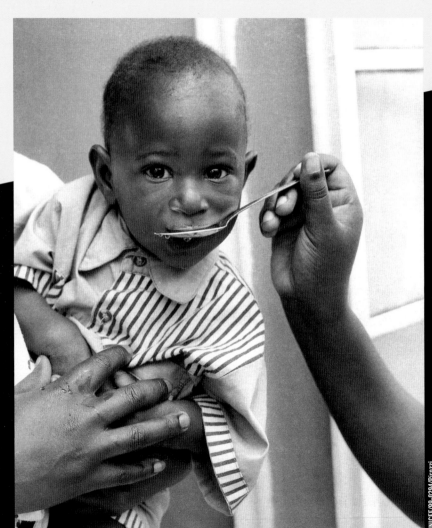

Why it is important to share and act on information about

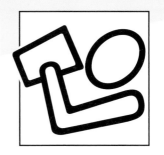

Diarrhoea

Diarrhoea kills over 1 million children every year through dehydration and malnutrition. Children are more likely than adults to die from diarrhoea because they become dehydrated more quickly. About 1 in every 200 children who contract diarrhoea will die from it.

Diarrhoea is caused by germs that are swallowed, especially germs from faeces. This happens most often where there is unsafe disposal of faeces, poor hygiene practices or a lack of clean drinking water, or when infants are not breastfed. Infants who are fed only breast-milk seldom get diarrhoea.

If families and communities work together, with support from governments and non-governmental organizations (NGOs), they can do much to prevent the conditions that cause diarrhoea.

Key Messages:

**What every family and community
has a right to know about**

Diarrhoea

1. Diarrhoea kills children by draining liquid from the body, thus dehydrating the child. As soon as diarrhoea starts, it is essential that the child be given extra fluids as well as regular foods and fluids.

2. A child's life is in danger if there are several watery stools within an hour or if there is blood in the faeces. Immediate help from a trained health worker is needed.

3. Breastfeeding can reduce the severity and frequency of diarrhoea.

4. A child with diarrhoea needs to continue eating regularly. While recovering from diarrhoea, the child needs at least an extra meal every day for at least two weeks.

FACTS FOR LIFE

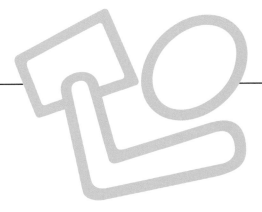

5. If the child is dehydrated with severe or persistent diarrhoea, only oral rehydration solution or medicines recommended by a trained health worker should be used. Other diarrhoea medicines are generally ineffective and could be harmful to the child.

6. To prevent diarrhoea, all faeces should be disposed of in a latrine or toilet or buried.

7. Good hygiene practices protect against diarrhoea. Hands should be thoroughly washed with soap and water or ash and water after contact with faeces, and before touching food or feeding children.

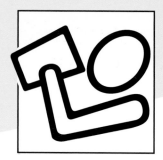

Diarrhoea

1. Diarrhoea kills children by draining liquid from the body, thus dehydrating the child. As soon as diarrhoea starts, it is essential that the child be given extra fluids as well as regular foods and fluids.

A child has diarrhoea when he or she passes three or more watery stools a day. The more numerous the watery stools, the more dangerous the diarrhoea.

Some people think that drinking liquids makes diarrhoea worse. *This is not true.* A child with diarrhoea should be given drinks as often as possible until the diarrhoea stops. Drinking lots of liquids helps to replace the fluids lost during diarrhoea.

Recommended drinks for a child with diarrhoea:

- breastmilk (mothers should breastfeed more often than usual)

- soups

- rice water

- fresh fruit juices

- weak tea with a little sugar

- coconut water

- clean water from a safe source. If there is a possibility the water is not clean, it should be purified by boiling or filtering.

- oral rehydration salts (ORS) mixed with the proper amount of clean water. (*See box on page 83.*)

To avoid dehydration, breastfed children should breast-feed as often as possible, and other children should drink the following amounts of liquids every time a watery stool is passed:

- for a child under the age of two years: between a quarter and a half of a large cup

- for a child aged two or older: between a half and a whole large cup.

Drinks should be given from a clean cup. A feeding bottle should never be used. It is difficult to clean bottles completely and unclean bottles can cause diarrhoea.

If the child vomits, the caregiver should wait for 10 minutes and then begin again to give the drink to the child slowly, small sips at a time.

The child should be given extra liquids until the diarrhoea has stopped.

Diarrhoea usually stops after three or four days. If it lasts longer than one week, caregivers should seek help from a trained health worker.

2. A child's life is in danger if there are several watery stools within an hour or if there is blood in the faeces. Immediate help from a trained health worker is needed.

Parents should immediately seek help from a trained health worker if the child:

- passes several watery stools in one or two hours

- passes blood in the faeces

- vomits frequently

- has a fever

- is extremely thirsty

- does not want to drink

- refuses to eat

- has sunken eyes

- looks weak or is lethargic

- has had diarrhoea for more than one week.

If the child has *any* of these signs, help from a trained health worker is needed urgently. In the meantime, the child should be given ORS solution or other liquids.

If the child passes several watery stools in one or two hours and vomits, there is cause for alarm – these are possible signs of cholera. Cholera can kill children in a matter of hours. Seek medical help immediately.

- Cholera can spread throughout the community quickly through contaminated water or food. Cholera usually occurs in situations where there is poor sanitation and overcrowding.

- There are four steps to be taken to limit the spread of cholera or diarrhoea:

  1. Dispose of all faeces in a latrine or toilet or bury them

  2. Wash hands with soap or ash and water after contact with faeces

  3. Use safe drinking water

  4. Wash, peel or cook all foods.

3. Breastfeeding can reduce the severity and frequency of diarrhoea.

Breastmilk is the best source of liquid and food for a young child with diarrhoea. It is nutritious and clean and helps fight illness and infections. An infant who is fed only breastmilk is unlikely to get diarrhoea.

Breastmilk prevents dehydration and malnutrition and helps replace lost fluids. Mothers are sometimes advised to give less breastmilk if a child has diarrhoea. *This advice is wrong.* Mothers should breastfeed more often than usual when the child has diarrhoea.

4. **A child with diarrhoea needs to continue eating regularly. While recovering from diarrhoea, the child needs at least an extra meal every day for at least two weeks.**

A child with diarrhoea loses weight and can quickly become malnourished. A child with diarrhoea needs all the food and fluid he or she can take. Food can help stop the diarrhoea and help the child recover more quickly.

A child with diarrhoea may not want to eat or may vomit, so feeding can be difficult. If the child is around six months of age or older, parents and caregivers should encourage the child to eat as often as possible, offering small amounts of soft, mashed foods or foods the child likes. These foods should contain a small amount of salt. Soft foods are easier to eat and contain more fluid than hard foods.

Recommended foods for a child with diarrhoea are well-mashed mixes of cereals and beans, fish, well-cooked meat, yogurt and fruits. One or two teaspoons of oil can be added to cereal and vegetables. Foods should be freshly prepared and given to the child five or six times a day.

After the diarrhoea stops, extra feeding is vital for a full recovery. At this time, the child needs to eat an extra meal a day, or breastfeed more every day, for at least two weeks. This will help the child replace the energy and nourishment lost due to diarrhoea.

A child is not fully recovered from diarrhoea until he or she is at least the same weight as when the illness began.

Vitamin A capsules and foods that contain vitamin A help a child recover from diarrhoea. Foods that contain vitamin A include breastmilk, liver, fish, dairy products, orange or yellow fruits and vegetables, and green leafy vegetables.

5. If the child is dehydrated with severe or persistent diarrhoea, only oral rehydration solution or medicines recommended by a trained health worker should be used. Other diarrhoea medicines are generally ineffective and could be harmful to the child.

Diarrhoea usually cures itself in a few days. The real danger is the loss of liquid and nutrients from the child's body, which can cause dehydration and malnutrition.

A child with diarrhoea should never be given any tablets, antibiotics or other medicines unless these have been prescribed by a trained health worker.

The best treatment for diarrhoea is to drink lots of liquids and oral rehydration salts (ORS) properly mixed with water.

If ORS packets are not available, dehydration can be treated by giving the child a drink made with four level teaspoons of sugar and half a level teaspoon of salt dissolved in one litre of clean water. Be very careful to mix the correct amounts, as too much sugar can make the diarrhoea worse, and too much salt can be extremely harmful to the child. If the mixture is made a little too diluted no harm can be done and there is very little loss of effectiveness.

Measles frequently causes severe diarrhoea. Immunizing children against measles prevents this cause of diarrhoea.

ORS solution
A special drink for diarrhoea

What is ORS?

ORS (oral rehydration salts) is a special combination of dry salts that, when properly mixed with safe water, can help rehydrate the body when a lot of fluid has been lost due to diarrhoea.

Where can ORS be obtained?

In most countries, ORS packets are available from health centres, pharmacies, markets and shops.

To make the ORS drink:

1. Put the contents of the ORS packet in a clean container. Check the packet for directions and add the correct amount of clean water. Too little water could make the diarrhoea worse.

2. Add water only. Do not add ORS to milk, soup, fruit juice or soft drinks. Do not add sugar.

3. Stir well, and feed it to the child from a clean cup. Do not use a bottle.

How much ORS drink to give?

Encourage the child to drink as much as possible.

A child under the age of two needs at least a quarter to a half of a large cup of the ORS drink after each watery stool.

A child aged two or older needs at least a half to a whole large cup of the ORS drink after each watery stool.

Diarrhoea usually stops in three or four days.

If it does not stop after one week, consult a trained health worker.

6. To prevent diarrhoea, all faeces should be disposed of in a latrine or toilet or buried.

Children and adults can swallow germs that cause diarrhoea if faeces touch the household's drinking water, food, hands, utensils or food preparation surfaces. Flies that settle on faeces and then on food also transmit the germs that cause diarrhoea. Covering food and drinking water protects them from flies.

All faeces, even those of infants and young children, carry germs and are therefore dangerous. If children defecate without using the latrine or toilet, their faeces should be cleaned up immediately and put down the toilet or buried. Keeping latrines and toilets clean prevents the spread of germs.

If there is no access to a toilet or latrine, adults and children should defecate away from houses, paths, water supplies and places where children play and then the faeces should be buried under a layer of soil.

In communities without toilets or latrines, the community should consider joining together to build such facilities.

Water sources should be kept clear of animal or human faeces.

7. Good hygiene practices protect against diarrhoea.

Hands should be thoroughly washed with soap and water or ash and water after contact with faeces, and before touching food or feeding children.

Hands should always be washed with soap and water or ash and water after defecating, after cleaning the baby's bottom, and immediately before feeding children, handling food or eating.

Young children frequently put their hands in their mouths, so it is important to keep the household area clean and to wash children's hands often with water and soap or ash, especially before giving them food.

Other hygiene measures can help to prevent diarrhoea:

● Food should be prepared and thoroughly cooked just before eating. Food left standing can collect germs that can cause diarrhoea. After two hours cooked foods are not safe unless they are kept very hot or very cold.

● All refuse should be buried, burned or safely disposed of to stop flies from spreading disease.

DIARRHOEA

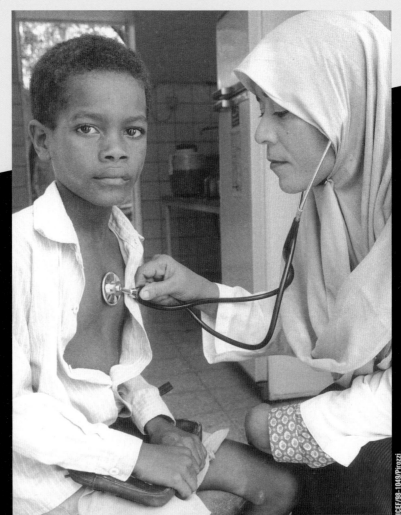

Why it is important to share and act on information about

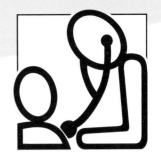

Coughs, Colds and More Serious Illnesses

Coughs, colds, sore throats and runny noses are common occurrences in the lives of children and usually are no cause for alarm.

In some cases, however, coughs and colds are danger signs of more serious illnesses such as pneumonia or tuberculosis. Respiratory infections killed some 2 million children under the age of five in the year 2000.

Key Messages:

What every family and community has a right to know about

Coughs, Colds and More Serious Illnesses

1. A child with a cough or cold should be kept warm and encouraged to eat and drink as much as possible.

2. Sometimes, coughs and colds are signs of a serious problem. A child who is breathing rapidly or with difficulty might have pneumonia, an infection of the lungs. This is a life-threatening disease and the child needs immediate treatment at a health facility.

3. Families can help prevent pneumonia by making sure that babies are exclusively breastfed for at least the first six months and that all children are well nourished and fully immunized.

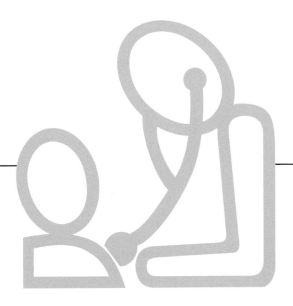

4. A child with a harsh cough needs immediate medical attention. The child may have tuberculosis, an infection in the lungs.

5. Children and pregnant women are particularly at risk when exposed to smoke from tobacco or cooking fires.

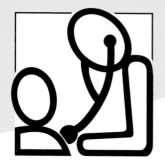

Coughs, Colds and More Serious Illnesses

1. A child with a cough or cold should be kept warm and encouraged to eat and drink as much as possible.

Babies and very young children lose their body heat easily. When they have a cough or cold they should be kept covered and warm.

Children with coughs, colds, runny noses or sore throats who are breathing normally can be treated at home and will recover without medicines. They need to be kept warm, but not overheated, and be given plenty to eat and drink. Medication should be used only if prescribed by a health worker.

A child with a fever should be sponged or bathed with cool but not cold water. In areas where malaria is common, the fever could be dangerous. The child should be checked by a health worker immediately.

The nose of a child with a cough or cold should be cleared often, especially before the child eats or goes to sleep. A moist atmosphere can make breathing easier, and it will help if the child breathes water vapour from a bowl of hot but not boiling water.

A breastfed child who has a cough or cold may have difficulty feeding. But breastfeeding helps to fight the illness and is important for the child's growth, so the mother should continue to breastfeed often. If a child cannot suckle, the breastmilk can be expelled into a clean cup and the child can then be fed from the cup.

Children who are not breastfed should be encouraged to eat or drink small amounts frequently. When the illness is over, the child should be given an extra meal every day for at least a week. The child is not fully recovered until he or she is at least the same weight as before the illness.

Coughs and colds spread easily. People with coughs and colds should avoid coughing, sneezing or spitting near children.

2. **Sometimes, coughs and colds are signs of a serious problem. A child who is breathing rapidly or with difficulty might have pneumonia, an infection of the lungs. This is a life-threatening disease and the child needs immediate treatment at a health facility.**

Most bouts of coughs, colds, sore throats and runny noses end without requiring medication. But sometimes these illnesses are signs of pneumonia, which usually requires antibiotics.

If a health worker provides antibiotics to treat the pneumonia, it is important to follow the instructions and give the child all the medicine for as long as the instructions say, even if the child seems better.

Many children die of pneumonia at home because their caregivers do not realize the seriousness of the illness and the need for immediate medical care. Millions of child deaths from pneumonia can be prevented if:

- parents and caregivers know that rapid and difficult breathing are danger signs, requiring urgent medical help

- parents and caregivers know where to get medical help

- medical help and low-cost antibiotics are readily available.

The child should be taken immediately to a health clinic or a trained health worker if any of the following are present:

FACTS FOR LIFE

- the child is breathing much more quickly than usual: for a child 2 to 12 months old – 50 breaths a minute or more; for a child 12 months to 5 years old – 40 breaths a minute or more

- the child is breathing with difficulty or gasping for air

- the lower part of the chest sucks in when the child breathes in, or it looks as though the stomach is moving up and down

- the child has had a cough for more than two weeks

- the child is unable to breastfeed or drink

- the child vomits frequently.

3. Families can help prevent pneumonia by making sure that babies are exclusively breastfed for at least the first six months and that all children are well nourished and fully immunized.

Breastfeeding helps to protect babies from pneumonia and other illnesses. It is important to give breastmilk alone for the first six months of a baby's life.

At any age, a child who is well fed is less likely to become seriously ill or die.

Vitamin A helps protect against severe respiratory disease and other illnesses and speeds recovery. Vitamin A is found in breastmilk, liver, red palm oil, fish, dairy products, eggs, some orange and yellow fruits and vegetables, and green leafy vegetables. Vitamin A supplements can also be given by a health worker.

Immunization should be completed before the child is one year old. The child will then be protected against measles, which can lead to pneumonia and other respiratory illnesses, including whooping cough and tuberculosis.

4. **A child with a harsh cough needs immediate medical attention. The child may have tuberculosis, an infection in the lungs.**

Tuberculosis is a serious disease that can kill a child or permanently damage the lungs. Families can help prevent tuberculosis if they ensure that children:

● are fully immunized – BCG immunization offers some protection against some forms of tuberculosis

● are kept away from anyone who has tuberculosis or has a cough with bloody sputum.

If the health worker provides special medications for tuberculosis, it is important to give the child all the medicine according to the instructions for as long as specified, even if the child seems better.

5. **Children and pregnant women are particularly at risk when exposed to smoke from tobacco or cooking fires.**

Children are more likely to get pneumonia and other breathing problems if they live in an environment with smoke.

Exposure to smoke can harm a child, even before birth. Pregnant women should not smoke or be exposed to smoke.

Tobacco use generally begins during adolescence. Adolescents are more likely to start smoking if the adults around them smoke, if tobacco advertising and promotion are common and if tobacco products are cheap and easily accessible. Adolescents should be encouraged to avoid smoking and to caution their friends about its dangers.

COUGHS, COLDS & MORE
SERIOUS ILLNESSES

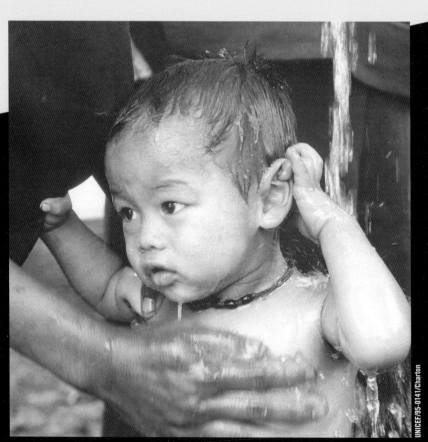

Why it is important to share and act on information about

Hygiene

More than half of all illnesses and deaths among young children are caused by germs that get into their mouths through food or water or dirty hands. Many of these germs come from human and animal faeces.

Many illnesses, especially diarrhoea, can be prevented by good hygiene practices: putting all faeces in a toilet or latrine; washing hands with soap and water or ash and water after defecating or handling children's faeces, and before feeding children or touching food; and ensuring that animal faeces are kept away from the house, paths, wells and children's play areas.

Everyone in the community needs to work together to build and use toilets and latrines, protect water sources, and safely dispose of waste water and garbage. It is important for governments to support communities by providing information on low-cost latrines and toilet facilities that all families can afford. In urban areas, government support is needed for low-cost sanitation and drainage systems, improved drinking water supply, and garbage collection.

Key Messages:

What every family and community has a right to know about

Hygiene

1. All faeces should be disposed of safely. Using a toilet or latrine is the best way.

2. All family members, including children, need to wash their hands thoroughly with soap and water or ash and water after contact with faeces, before touching food, and before feeding children.

3. Washing the face with soap and water every day helps to prevent eye infections. In some parts of the world, eye infections can lead to trachoma, which can cause blindness.

4. Only use water that is from a safe source or is purified. Water containers need to be kept covered to keep the water clean.

FACTS FOR LIFE

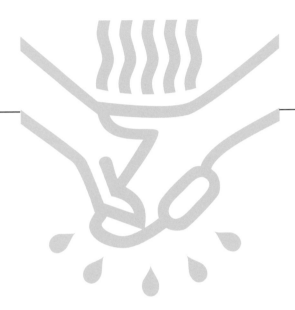

5. Raw or leftover food can be dangerous. Raw food should be washed or cooked. Cooked food should be eaten without delay or thoroughly reheated.

6. Food, utensils and food preparation surfaces should be kept clean. Food should be stored in covered containers.

7. Safe disposal of all household refuse helps prevent illness.

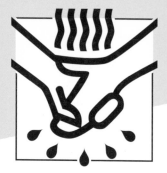

Hygiene

1. All faeces should be disposed of safely. Using a toilet or latrine is the best way.

Many illnesses, especially diarrhoea, come from germs found in human faeces. If the germs get into water or onto food, hands, utensils or surfaces used for preparing and serving food, they can be swallowed and cause illness.

The single most important action to prevent the spread of germs is to dispose of all faeces – both human and animal – safely. Human faeces need to be put down a toilet or latrine. The latrine needs to be kept clean. Animal faeces need to be kept away from the house, paths and areas where children play.

If it is not possible to use a toilet or latrine, everyone should always defecate well away from houses, paths, water sources and places where children play. The faeces should be buried immediately.

All faeces, even those of infants, carry germs and are therefore dangerous. If children defecate without using a toilet, latrine or potty, their faeces should be cleaned up immediately and put down the latrine or buried.

Latrines and toilets need to be cleaned frequently. Latrines should be kept covered and toilets should be flushed.

Local governments and NGOs often can help communities build sanitary latrines by giving advice on the design and construction of low-cost latrines.

2. **All family members, including children, need to wash their hands thoroughly with soap and water or ash and water after contact with faeces, before touching food, and before feeding children.**

Washing the hands with soap and water or ash and water removes germs. Rinsing the fingers with water is not enough – both hands need to be rubbed with soap or ash. This helps to stop germs and dirt from getting onto food or into the mouth. Washing the hands can also prevent infection with worms. Soap and water or ash and water should be placed conveniently near the latrine or toilet.

● It is especially important to wash the hands after defecating and after cleaning the bottom of a baby or child who has just defecated. It is also important to wash hands after handling animals and raw foods.

● Hands should always be washed before preparing, serving or eating food, and before feeding children. Children should be taught to wash both hands after defecating and before eating to help protect them from illness.

Children often put their hands into their mouths, so it is important to wash a child's hands often, especially after they have been playing in dirt or with animals.

Children are easily infected with worms, which deplete the body's nutrients. Worms and their eggs can be found in human and animal faeces and urine, in surface water and soil, and in poorly cooked meat. Children should not play near the latrine, toilet or defecation areas. Shoes should be worn near latrines to prevent worms from entering the body through the skin of the feet.

● Children living in areas where worms are common should be treated two to three times per year with a recommended antihelmenthic medication.

HYGIENE

3. **Washing the face with soap** and water every day helps to prevent eye infections. In some parts of the world, eye infections can lead to trachoma, which can cause blindness.

A dirty face attracts flies, spreading the germs they carry from person to person. The eyes may become sore or infected and vision may be impaired or lost if the eyes are not kept clean and healthy.

If the eyes are healthy, the white part is clear, the eyes are moist and shiny, and vision is sharp. If the eyes are extremely dry or very red and sore, if there is a discharge or if there is difficulty seeing, then the child should be examined by a health worker as soon as possible.

---

4. **Only use water that is** from a safe source or is purified. Water containers need to be kept covered to keep the water clean.

Families have fewer illnesses when they have an adequate supply of clean water and know how to keep it free of germs.

If the water is not clean it can be purified by boiling or filtering.

Clean water sources include properly constructed and maintained piped systems, tube-wells, protected dug wells and springs. Water from unsafe sources – such as ponds, rivers, open tanks and step-wells – can be made safer by boiling. Water should be stored in a covered container to keep it clean.

Families and communities can protect their water supply by:

- keeping wells covered and installing a handpump

- disposing of faeces and waste water (especially from latrines and household cleaning) well away from any water source used for cooking, drinking or washing

- building latrines at least 15 metres away and downhill from a water source

- always keeping buckets, ropes and jars used to collect and store water as clean as possible by storing them in a clean place, rather than on the ground

- keeping animals away from drinking water sources and family living areas

- avoiding the use of pesticides or chemicals anywhere near a water source.

Families can keep water clean in the home by:

- storing drinking water in a clean, covered container

- avoid touching clean water with unclean hands

- taking water out of the container with a clean ladle or cup

- having a tap on the water container

- not allowing anyone to put their hands into the container or to drink directly from it

- keeping animals away from stored water.

If there is uncertainty about the safety of the drinking water, local authorities should be consulted.

---

5. Raw or leftover food can be dangerous. Raw food should be washed or cooked. Cooked food should be eaten without delay or thoroughly reheated.

Cooking food thoroughly kills germs. Food, especially meat and poultry, should be cooked all the way through.

Germs grow quickly in warm food. Food should be eaten as soon as possible after cooking so it does not have time to collect germs.

- If food has to be kept for more than two hours, it should be kept either very hot or very cool.

- If cooked food is saved for another meal, it should be covered to keep off flies and insects and then thoroughly reheated before being eaten.

HYGIENE

- Yogurt and sour porridge are good to use in meals because their acid prevents the growth of germs.

Raw food, especially poultry and seafood, usually contains germs. Cooked food can collect germs if it touches raw food. So raw and cooked foods should always be kept away from each other. Knives, chopping boards and surfaces where food is prepared should always be cleaned after preparing raw food.

- Breastmilk is the safest milk for infants and young children. Animal milk that is freshly boiled or pasteurized is safer than unboiled milk.

- Expressed breastmilk can be stored at room temperature for up to eight hours in a clean, covered container.

- Special care should be taken with preparing food for infants and small children. Their food should be freshly made and not left standing, if possible.

- Fruit and vegetables should be peeled or washed thoroughly with clean water, especially if they are to be given raw to babies or small children. Chemicals such as pesticides and herbicides cannot be seen on fruit and vegetables but nonetheless can be dangerous.

6. Food, utensils and food preparation surfaces should be kept clean. Food should be stored in covered containers.

Germs on food can be swallowed and cause illness. To protect food from germs:

- food preparation surfaces should be kept clean

- knives, cooking utensils, pots and plates should be kept clean and covered

- cloths for cleaning dishes or pans should be washed thoroughly every day and dried in the sun. Plates, utensils and pans should be washed immediately after eating and put on a rack to dry

- food should be kept in covered containers to protect it from insects and animals

- feeding bottles or teats should not be used because they can contain germs that cause diarrhoea unless they are cleaned each time with boiling water. Children should be breastfed or fed from a clean, open cup.

7. Safe disposal of all household refuse helps prevent illness.

Germs can be spread by flies, cockroaches, rats and mice, which thrive in refuse such as food scraps and peelings from fruit and vegetables.

If there is no community-wide collection of garbage, each family needs a garbage pit where household refuse is buried or burned every day.

Keeping the household and nearby areas clean and free of faeces, refuse and waste water can help prevent disease. Household waste water can be disposed of safely by making a soak pit or a channel to the kitchen garden or to the field.

Chemicals such as pesticides and herbicides can be very dangerous if even small quantities get into the water supply or onto food, hands or feet. Clothes and containers used when handling chemicals should not be washed near a household water source.

Pesticides and other chemicals should not be used around the household or near a water source. Chemicals should not be stored in or near drinking water containers or near food. Never store food or water in pesticide or fertilizer containers.

HYGIENE

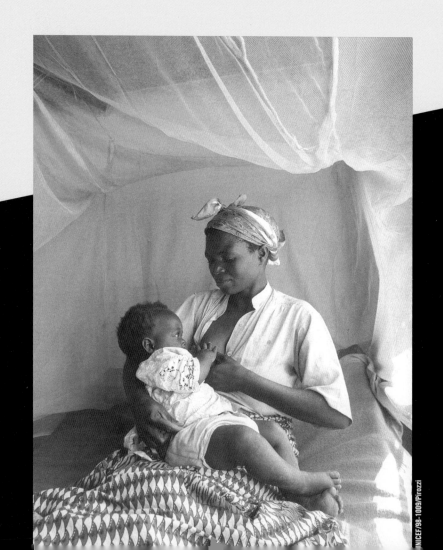

Why it is important to share and act on information about

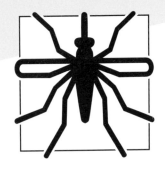

Malaria

Malaria is a serious disease spread through mosquito bites. Each year, there are 300 million to 500 million cases of malaria throughout the world and about 1 million child deaths. In areas where malaria is common, it can be the leading cause of death and poor growth among young children.

Malaria is also particularly dangerous for pregnant women. It causes severe anaemia, miscarriages, stillbirths, low birthweight and maternal death.

Many lives can be saved by the prevention and early treatment of malaria.

Key Messages:

What every family and community has a right to know about

Malaria

1. Malaria is transmitted through mosquito bites. Sleeping under a mosquito net treated with a recommended insecticide is the best way to prevent mosquito bites.

2. Wherever malaria is common, children are in danger. A child with a fever should be examined immediately by a trained health worker and receive an appropriate antimalarial treatment as soon as possible.

3. Malaria is very dangerous for pregnant women. Wherever malaria is common, pregnant women should prevent malaria by taking antimalarial tablets recommended by a health worker.

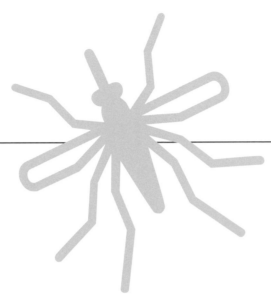

4. A child suffering or recovering from malaria needs plenty of liquids and food.

5. Families and communities can prevent malaria by taking action to stop mosquitoes from breeding.

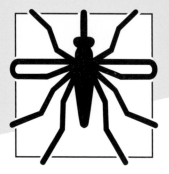

Malaria

1. Malaria is transmitted through mosquito bites. Sleeping under a mosquito net treated with a recommended insecticide is the best way to prevent mosquito bites.

All members of the community should be protected against mosquito bites, particularly young children and pregnant women, and especially between sunset and sunrise when mosquitos are most active.

Mosquito nets, curtains or mats that are dipped in a recommended insecticide kill mosquitoes that land on them. Special, permanently treated mats should be used, or nets, curtains or mats that are dipped in insecticide regularly. Usually, the nets need to be re-treated when the rains begin, at least every six months, and after every third wash. Trained health workers can advise on safe insecticides and re-treatment schedules.

Babies and other small children should sleep under a treated mosquito net. If the nets are expensive, the family should buy at least one big net, which the small children can sleep under. Breastfed babies should sleep with their mothers under a net.

Treated mosquito nets should be used throughout the year, even during times when there are fewer mosquitoes.

If mosquito nets cannot be used, other actions can help:

● curtains, cloths or mats impregnated with a recommended insecticide can be hung over doors and windows

- screens can be put on doors and windows

- mosquito coils or other fumigants can be used

- clothing that covers the arms and legs (long sleeves and long pants or skirts) can be worn as soon as it begins to get dark. This is especially important for children and pregnant women.

2. Wherever malaria is common, children are in danger. A child with a fever should be examined immediately by a trained health worker and receive an appropriate antimalarial treatment as soon as possible.

Malaria should be suspected if anyone in the family has a fever, or if young children refuse to eat or have vomiting, drowsiness or fits.

A child with a fever believed to be caused by malaria needs to be given immediate antimalarial treatment as recommended by a health worker. If children with a malarial fever are not treated within a day, they might die. A health worker can advise on what type of treatment is best and how long it should continue.

A child with malaria needs to take the full course of treatment, even if the fever disappears rapidly. If the treatment is not completed, the malaria could become more severe and difficult to cure.

If the malaria symptoms continue after treatment, the child should be taken to a health centre or hospital for help. The problem may be:

- the child is not receiving enough medicine

- the child has an illness other than malaria

- the malaria is resistant to the medicine, and another medicine is needed.

Children with a fever should be kept cool for as long as the fever persists by:

- sponging or bathing with cool (not cold) water

- covering the child with only a few clothes or one blanket.

---

3. Malaria is very dangerous for pregnant women. Wherever malaria is common, pregnant women should prevent malaria by taking antimalarial tablets recommended by a health worker.

Pregnant women are more likely to suffer from malaria than other women. The disease is more dangerous during pregnancy, especially during the first pregnancy. It can cause severe anaemia ('thin blood'), miscarriage, premature birth or stillbirth. Babies born to mothers who have had malaria during pregnancy will probably be underweight and therefore more vulnerable to infection or death during their first year.

Pregnant women should take antimalarial tablets during pregnancy where recommended.

Not all antimalarial tablets are safe to take during pregnancy. The health worker will know which antimalarial tablets are best.

Pregnant women need to sleep under mosquito nets that are regularly treated with insecticide to prevent mosquito bites.

Pregnant women with signs and symptoms of malaria must be treated adequately and immediately to prevent death.

Pregnant women who become ill with malaria should ask a health worker about iron and vitamin A supplements.

4. A child suffering or recovering from malaria needs plenty of liquids and food.

Malaria burns up energy, and the child loses a lot of body fluids through sweating. The child should be offered food and drink frequently to help prevent malnutrition and dehydration.

Frequent breastfeeding prevents dehydration and helps the child fight infections, including malaria. Children with malaria should be breastfed as often as possible.

Frequent malarial infection can slow children's growth and brain development and is likely to cause anaemia. A child who has had several bouts of malaria should be checked for anaemia.

5. Families and communities can prevent malaria by taking action to stop mosquitoes from breeding.

Mosquitoes breed wherever there is still water – for example, in ponds, swamps, puddles, pits, drains and in the moisture on long grass and bushes. They can also breed along the edges of streams and in water containers, tanks and rice fields.

The number of mosquitoes can be reduced by:

- filling in or draining places where water collects
- covering water containers or tanks
- clearing bushes around houses.

Malaria affects the whole community. Everyone can work together to reduce the breeding places for mosquitoes and to organize regular treatment of mosquito nets with insecticide. Communities should ask all health workers and political leaders in their regions to help them prevent and control malaria.

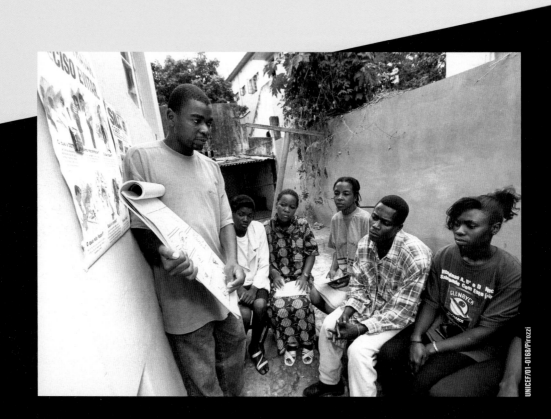

Why it is important to share and act on information about

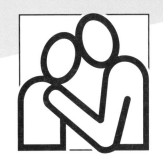

HIV/AIDS

People in every country of the world are affected by AIDS (acquired immune deficiency syndrome). HIV/AIDS is becoming more of a global crisis every day. At present, 40 million adults and children are living with HIV/AIDS, and at least 10.4 million children currently under the age of 15 have lost their mother or both parents to AIDS.

The disease increasingly affects young people. Of the 5 million new infections in 2001, approximately half are among young people between the ages of 15 and 24. Young women are especially vulnerable. An estimated 11.8 million young people are living with HIV/AIDS – 7.3 million young women and 4.5 million young men.

AIDS is caused by the human immunodeficiency virus (HIV). HIV damages the body's defences against other diseases. Medication can help people with HIV/AIDS live longer, but the disease so far has no vaccine or cure.

Prevention is the most effective strategy against the spread of HIV/AIDS. Every person in every country should know how to avoid getting and spreading the disease.

Condoms can save lives by preventing the sexual transmission of HIV. Access to testing and counselling must be given high priority in every country. Everyone has the right to voluntary and confidential counselling and testing for HIV/AIDS and the right to be protected from discrimination of any kind related to her or his HIV/AIDS status.

For those living with or affected by HIV/AIDS, care and compassion are needed. Measures should be taken to remove the social, cultural and political barriers that might block access to HIV/AIDS services and programmes.

Key Messages:

What every family and community has a right to know about

HIV/AIDS

1. AIDS is an incurable but preventable disease. HIV, the virus that causes AIDS, spreads through unprotected sex (intercourse without a condom), transfusions of unscreened blood, contaminated needles and syringes (most often those used for injecting drugs), and from an infected woman to her child during pregnancy, childbirth or breastfeeding.

2. All people, including children, are at risk for HIV/AIDS. Everyone needs information and education about the disease and access to condoms to reduce this risk.

3. Anyone who suspects that he or she might be infected with HIV should contact a health worker or an HIV/AIDS centre to receive confidential counselling and testing.

4. The risk of getting HIV through sex can be reduced if people don't have sex, if they reduce the number of sex partners, if uninfected partners have sex only with each other, or if people have safer sex – sex without penetration or while using a condom. Correct and consistent use of condoms can save lives by preventing the spread of HIV.

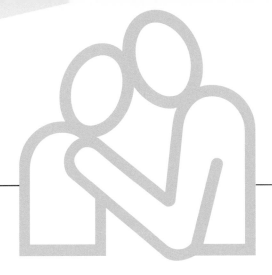

5. Girls are especially vulnerable to HIV infection and need support to protect themselves and be protected against unwanted and unsafe sex.

6. Parents and teachers can help young people protect themselves from HIV/AIDS by talking with them about how to avoid getting and spreading the disease, including the correct and consistent use of male or female condoms.

7. HIV infection can be passed from a mother to her child during pregnancy or childbirth or through breastfeeding. Pregnant women or new mothers who are infected with HIV, or suspect that they are infected, should consult a qualified health worker to seek testing and counselling.

8. HIV can be spread by unsterilized needles or syringes, most often those used for injecting drugs. Used razor blades, knives or tools that cut or pierce the skin also carry some risk of spreading HIV.

9. People who have a sexually transmitted infection (STI) are at greater risk of getting HIV and of spreading HIV to others. People with STIs should seek prompt treatment and avoid sexual intercourse or practice safer sex (non-penetrative sex or sex using a condom).

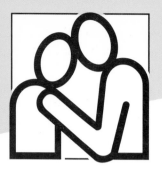

HIV/AIDS

1. AIDS is an incurable but preventable disease. HIV, the virus that causes AIDS, spreads through unprotected sex (intercourse without a condom), transfusions of unscreened blood, contaminated needles and syringes (most often those used for injecting drugs), and from an infected woman to her child during pregnancy, childbirth or breastfeeding.

AIDS is caused by the human immunodeficiency virus (HIV), which damages the body's defence system.

People infected with HIV usually live for years without any signs of the disease. They may look and feel healthy, but they can still pass on the virus to others.

AIDS is the late stage of HIV infection. People who have AIDS grow weaker because their bodies lose the ability to fight off illnesses. In adults, AIDS develops 7 to 10 years after infection, on average. In young children it usually develops much faster. AIDS is not curable, but new medicines can help people with AIDS live healthier for longer periods.

In most cases, HIV is passed from one person to another through unprotected sexual intercourse, during which the semen, vaginal fluid or blood of an infected person passes into the body of another person.

HIV can also pass from one person to another through the use of unsterilized needles and syringes (most often those used for injecting drugs), razor blades, knives or other instruments for injecting, cutting or piercing the body, and through transfusions of infected blood. All blood for transfusions should be screened for HIV.

It is *not* possible to get HIV/AIDS from touching those who are infected. Hugging, shaking hands, coughing and sneezing will not spread the disease. HIV/AIDS cannot be transmitted through toilet seats, telephones, plates, glasses, eating utensils, towels, bed linen, swimming pools or public baths. HIV/AIDS is *not* spread by mosquitos or other insects.

2. All people, including children, are at risk for HIV/AIDS. Everyone needs information and education about the disease and access to condoms to reduce this risk.

Babies and young children living with HIV/AIDS have special needs for good nutrition, immunization and regular health care to avoid complications from common childhood illnesses, which can be fatal. If the child is infected, it is likely that the mother, and probably also the father, is infected. Home care visits might be needed.

In countries with high rates of HIV infection, children are not only at risk of being infected, but they are also affected by the impact of HIV/AIDS on their families and communities.

● If children lose parents, teachers and caregivers to HIV/AIDS, they will need help in understanding what is happening and dealing with their loss and grief.

● Orphaned children might have to assume responsibilities as the head of the household and will undoubtedly face great economic difficulties. If orphaned children are cared for by others, then that family's limited resources must stretch to accommodate the additional needs of these children.

● Children living with HIV/AIDS or with families affected by HIV/AIDS may be stigmatized or isolated from their community and denied access to health services and school. Good-quality training on HIV/AIDS for teachers and peer educators can increase understanding and compassion and lessen discrimination.

Efforts should be made to keep HIV/AIDS-affected families together. Efforts should also be made to avoid institutionalizing orphaned children. Orphans are less traumatized if they are cared for by the extended family or the community.

Few young people receive the accurate and appropriate information they need. School-aged children should be provided with age-appropriate information on HIV/AIDS and life skills *before* they become sexually active. Education at this stage has been shown to delay sexual activity and to teach responsibility.

Children living in institutions, on the streets or in refugee camps are at even greater risk of being infected with HIV than are other children. Support services need to be provided accordingly.

---

3. Anyone who suspects that he or she might be infected with HIV should contact a health worker or an HIV/AIDS centre to receive confidential counselling and testing.

HIV counselling and testing can help in the early detection of HIV infection and in enabling those who are infected to get the support services they need, manage other infectious diseases they might have, and learn about living with HIV/AIDS and how to avoid infecting others. Counselling and testing can also help those not infected to remain uninfected through education about safer sex.

If the result of an HIV/AIDS test is negative, this means the person tested is not infected or it is too early to detect the virus. The HIV blood test may not detect infection up to the first six months. The test should be repeated six months after any possible exposure to HIV infection. Since an infected person can transmit the virus at any time, it is important to use a condom during sex or to avoid penetration.

Families and communities should demand and support confidential HIV/AIDS counselling, testing and information to help protect adults and children from the disease.

FACTS FOR LIFE

An HIV/AIDS test can help couples decide whether to have children. If one partner is infected, he or she could infect the other while attempting to conceive.

It is possible to stop HIV from spreading to the next generation if young people know the facts about HIV transmission, abstain from sex, and have access to condoms.

4. The risk of getting HIV through sex can be reduced if people don't have sex, if they reduce the number of sex partners, if uninfected partners have sex only with each other, or if people have safer sex – sex without penetration or while using a condom. Correct and consistent use of condoms can save lives by preventing the spread of HIV.

Mutual fidelity between two uninfected partners protects them both from HIV/AIDS.

The more sex partners people have, the greater the risk that one of them will have HIV/AIDS and pass it on. However, anyone can have HIV/AIDS – it is not restricted to those who have many sex partners.

● A blood test is the most accurate way to tell if someone is infected with HIV. An infected person may look completely healthy.

Unless partners have sex only with each other and are sure that they are both uninfected, they should practice safer sex. Safer sex means non-penetrative sex (where the penis does not enter the mouth, vagina or rectum) or the use of a new latex condom for every act of intercourse. (Latex condoms are less likely to break or leak than animal-skin condoms or the thinner 'more sensitive' condoms.) Condoms should never be re-used.

● A condom should always be used during all penetrative sex unless it is absolutely certain that both partners are free of HIV infection. A person can become infected through even one occasion of unprotected penetrative sex (sex without a condom).

- Condoms must be used for vaginal and anal intercourse for HIV prevention.

Condoms with lubrication (slippery liquid or gel) already on them are less likely to tear during handling or use. If the condom is not lubricated enough, a 'water-based' lubricant, such as silicone or glycerine, should be added. If such lubricants are not available, saliva can be used. Lubricants made from oil or petroleum (cooking oil or shortening, mineral or baby oil, petroleum jellies such as Vaseline, most lotions) should never be used because they can damage the condom. A well-lubricated condom is absolutely essential for protection during anal intercourse.

- HIV can be transmitted through oral sex. Hence, a condom should be used on a man, and a flat piece of latex or 'dam' on a woman.

Because most sexually transmitted infections (STIs) can be spread through genital contact, a condom should be used before genital contact begins.

Sex without penetration is another way to have safer sex that greatly decreases the risk of getting infected with HIV (though even this does not protect against all STIs).

A safe alternative to the male condom is the female condom. The female condom is a soft, loose-fitting polyurethane sheath that lines the vagina. It has a soft ring at each end. The ring at the closed end is used to put the device inside the vagina and to hold it in place during sex. The other ring stays outside the vagina and partly covers the labia. Before sex begins, the woman inserts the female condom with her fingers. Unlike the male condom, the female condom can be used with any lubricant – whether water-based, oil-based or petroleum-based – because it is made from polyurethane.

Drinking alcohol or taking drugs interferes with judgement. Even those who understand the risks of AIDS and the importance of safer sex may become careless after drinking or using drugs.

5. Girls are especially vulnerable to HIV infection and need support to protect themselves and be protected against unwanted and unsafe sex.

In many countries, HIV rates are much higher among teenage girls than teenage boys. Teenage girls are more susceptible to HIV infection because:

- young girls may not understand the risk or may be unable to protect themselves from sexual advances

- their vaginal membranes are thinner and more susceptible to infection than those of mature women

- they are sometimes targeted by older men who seek young women with little or no sexual experience because they are less likely to be infected.

Girls and women have the right to refuse unwanted and unprotected sex. Parents and teachers should discuss this issue with girls and boys to make them aware of girls' and women's rights, to teach boys to respect girls as equals, and to help girls avoid or defend themselves against unwanted sexual advances.

6. Parents and teachers can help young people protect themselves from HIV/AIDS by talking with them about how to avoid getting and spreading the disease, including the correct and consistent use of male or female condoms.

Young people need to understand the risks of HIV/AIDS. Parents, teachers, health workers, guardians or the person in the community in charge of rites of passage can warn young people about the risk of HIV/AIDS, other STIs and unplanned pregnancy.

It can be awkward to discuss sexual issues with young people. One way to begin the discussion with school-aged children is to ask them what they have heard about HIV/AIDS. If any of their information is wrong, take the opportunity to provide them with the correct information. Talking with and listening to young people is very important. If the parent is uncomfortable with the discussion, he or she can ask a teacher, a relative or someone who is good at discussing sensitive issues for advice on how to talk to the child about this.

Young people need to be informed that there is no vaccination and no cure for HIV/AIDS. They need to understand that prevention is the only protection against the disease. Young people also need to be empowered to refuse sex.

Children need to know that they do not run the risk of getting HIV from ordinary social contact with children or adults who are HIV infected.

Those living with HIV/AIDS need care and support. Young people can help by showing them compassion.

7. HIV infection can be passed from a mother to her child during pregnancy or childbirth or through breastfeeding. Pregnant women or new mothers who are infected with HIV, or suspect that they are infected, should consult a qualified health worker to seek testing and counselling.

The most effective way to reduce transmission of HIV from the mother to the child is to prevent HIV infection in women.

Empowering women and promoting safer sex, condom use and better detection and treatment of STIs can reduce HIV infection in women. If a woman discovers that she is HIV positive, she needs emotional support and counselling to help her make decisions and plan for her future. Community support groups and NGOs can support women in making these decisions.

Pregnant women need to know:

- that treatment with specified medicines during pregnancy can greatly reduce the risk of passing the infection to the infant

- that special care during pregnancy and delivery can reduce the risks of passing the infection to the infant.

New mothers need to know the different options for feeding their infants and the related risks. Health workers can assist in identifying a feeding method that can maximize the infant's chance of growing up healthy and free of HIV.

Babies born to women who have not received medication and are infected with HIV have about a 1-in-3 chance of being born with HIV. More than two thirds of the infants infected with HIV may die before they are five years old.

8. HIV can be spread by unsterilized needles or syringes, most often those used for injecting drugs. Used razor blades, knives or tools that cut or pierce the skin also carry some risk of spreading HIV.

An unsterilized needle or syringe can pass HIV from one person to another. Nothing should be used to pierce a person's skin unless it has been sterilized.

People who inject themselves with drugs or have unprotected sex with injecting drug users are at high risk of becoming infected with HIV. People who inject drugs should always use a clean needle and syringe, and never use another person's needle or syringe.

Injections should be given only by a trained health worker. For each child or adult being immunized, a new or fully sterilized needle and syringe should be used.

Sharing needles and syringes with anyone, including family members, may transmit HIV or other life-threatening diseases. No one should share needles or syringes. Parents should ask the health worker to use a new or sterilized needle for every person.

Any kind of cut using an unsterilized object such as a razor or knife can transmit HIV. The cutting instrument must be fully sterilized for each person, including family members, or rinsed with bleach and/or boiling water.

Any instrument that is used to cut a newborn's umbilical cord must be sterilized. Particular care should be taken when handling the placenta and any blood from the delivery. Protective (latex) gloves should be used if available.

Equipment for dental treatment, tattooing, facial marking, ear piercing and acupuncture is not safe unless the equipment is sterilized for each person. The person performing the procedure should take care to avoid any contact with blood during the procedure.

9. People who have a sexually transmitted infection (STI) are at greater risk of getting HIV and of spreading HIV to others. People with STIs should seek prompt treatment and avoid sexual intercourse or practice safer sex (non-penetrative sex or sex using a condom).

Sexually transmitted infections (STIs) are infections that are spread through sexual contact, either through the exchange of body fluids (semen, vaginal fluid or blood) or by contact with the skin of the genital area (particularly if there are lesions such as blisters, abrasions or cuts, often caused by the STI itself).

STIs often cause serious physical suffering and damage.

Any STI, such as gonorrhoea or syphilis, can increase the risk of catching or transmitting HIV. Persons suffering from an STI have a 5 to 10 times higher risk of becoming infected with HIV if they have unprotected sexual intercourse with an HIV-infected person.

● Correct and consistent use of latex condoms when engaging in sexual intercourse – vaginal, anal or oral – can greatly reduce the spread of most STIs, including HIV.

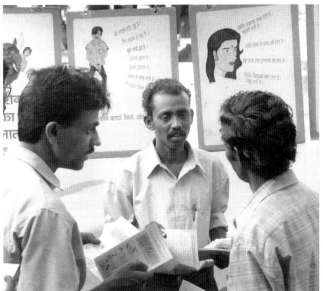

UNICEF/00-0110/Lewnes

- People who suspect that they have an STI should seek prompt treatment from a health worker in order to be diagnosed and get treatment. They should avoid sexual intercourse or practice safer sex (non-penetrative sex or sex using a condom). If found to have an STI, they should tell their partner. If both partners are not treated for an STI, they will continue infecting each other with the STI. Most STIs are curable.

A man infected with an STI may have pain or discomfort while urinating; discharge from his penis; or sores, blisters, bumps and rashes on the genitals or inside of the mouth. A woman infected with an STI may have discharge from the vagina that has a strange colour or bad smell, pain or itching around the genital area, and pain or unexpected bleeding from the vagina during or after intercourse. More severe infections can cause fever, pain in the abdomen, and infertility. However, many STIs in women produce no symptoms at all – and some STIs in men also may not have any noticeable symptoms.

Also, not every problem in the genital area is an STI. There are some infections, such as candidiasis and urinary tract infections, that are not spread by sexual intercourse but cause great discomfort in the genital area.

The traditional method of diagnosing STIs is by laboratory tests. However, these are often unavailable or too expensive. Since 1990, WHO has recommended 'syndromic management' of STIs in people with symptoms of STI. The main features of syndromic management are:

- classification of the main germs by the clinical syndromes produced

- use of flow charts derived from this classification to manage a particular syndrome

- treatment for all important causes of the syndrome

- notification and treatment of sex partners

- no expensive laboratory procedures.

The syndromic approach using flow charts offers accessible and immediate treatment that is cost-effective and efficient.

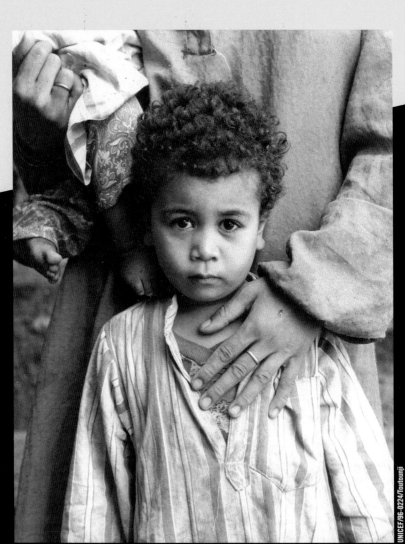

Why it is important to share and act on information about

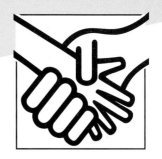

Injury Prevention

Every year, 750,000 children die from injuries. Another 400 million are seriously hurt. Many injuries lead to permanent disability and brain damage. Injuries are a major cause of death and disability among young children.

The most common injuries are falls, burns, drowning and road accidents. Most of these injuries happen in or near the home. Almost all can be prevented. Many would be less serious if parents knew what to do when an injury happens.

Key Messages:

What every family and community has a right to know about

Injury Prevention

1. Many serious injuries can be prevented if parents and caretakers watch young children carefully and keep their environment safe.

2. Children should be kept away from fires, cooking stoves, lamps, matches and electrical appliances.

3. Young children like to climb. Stairs, balconies, roofs, windows and play areas should be made secure to protect children from falling.

4. Knives, scissors, sharp or pointed objects and broken glass can cause serious injuries. These objects should be kept out of children's reach.

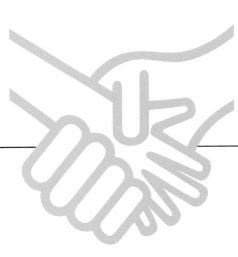

5. Young children like to put things in their mouths. Small objects should be kept out of their reach to prevent choking.

6. Poisons, medicines, bleach, acid, and liquid fuels such as paraffin (kerosene) should never be stored in drinking bottles. All such liquids and poisons should be kept in clearly marked containers out of children's sight and reach.

7. Children can drown in less than two minutes and in a very small amount of water. They should never be left alone when they are in or near water.

8. Children under five years old are particularly at risk on the roads. They should always have someone with them and they should be taught safe road behaviour as soon as they can walk.

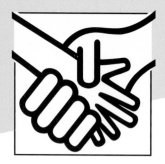

Injury Prevention

---

1. Many serious injuries can be prevented if parents and caretakers watch young children carefully and keep their environment safe.

Children between 18 months and four years old are at high risk of death and serious injuries. Most of these injuries happen in the home. Almost all can be prevented.

The main causes of injuries in the home:

- burns from fires, stoves, ovens, cooking pots, hot foods, boiling water, steam, hot fats, paraffin lamps, irons and electrical appliances

- cuts from broken glass, knives, scissors or axes

- falls from cots, windows, tables and stairs

- choking on small objects such as coins, buttons or nuts

- poisoning from paraffin (kerosene), insecticide, bleach and detergents

- electrical shock from touching broken electrical appliances or wires, or poking sticks or knives into electric outlets.

Anything that may be dangerous for active young children should be stored safely away, out of their reach.

Children should never be expected to work long hours or to do work that is hazardous or interferes with schooling. Children must be protected from heavy labour, dangerous tools and exposure to poisonous chemicals.

2. Children should be kept away from fires, cooking stoves, lamps, matches and electrical appliances.

Burns and scalds are among the most common causes of serious injury among young children. Children need to be prevented from touching cooking stoves, boiling water, hot food and hot irons. Burns often cause serious injury and permanent scarring, and some are fatal. The great majority of these are preventable.

Burns can be prevented by:

- keeping young children away from fires, matches and cigarettes

- keeping stoves on a flat, raised surface out of the reach of children. If an open cooking fire is used, it should be made on a raised mound of clay, not directly on the ground.

- turning the handles of all cooking pots away from the reach of children

- keeping petrol, paraffin, lamps, matches, candles, lighters, hot irons and electric cords out of the reach of young children.

Children can be seriously injured if they put their fingers or other objects into electric sockets. Power sockets should be covered to prevent access.

Electric wires should be kept out of children's reach. Bare electric wires are particularly dangerous.

3. **Young children like to climb. Stairs, balconies, roofs, windows and play areas should be made secure to protect children from falling.**

Falls are a common cause of bruises, broken bones and serious head injuries. Serious falls can be prevented by:

- discouraging children from climbing onto unsafe places

- using railings to guard stairs, windows or balconies

- keeping the home clean and well lit.

4. **Knives, scissors, sharp or pointed objects and broken glass can cause serious injuries. These objects should be kept out of children's reach.**

Broken glass can cause serious cuts, loss of blood and infected wounds. Glass bottles should be kept out of the reach of young children, and the house and play area should be kept free of broken glass. Young children should be taught not to touch broken glass; older children should be taught to dispose of any broken glass safely.

Knives, razors and scissors should be kept out of the reach of young children. Older children should be trained to handle them safely.

Sharp metal objects, machinery and rusty cans can cause badly infected wounds. Children's play areas should be kept clear of these objects. Household refuse, including broken bottles and old cans, should be disposed of safely.

Other injuries around the home can be prevented by teaching children the dangers of throwing stones or other sharp objects and playing with knives or scissors.

5.
Young children like to put things in their mouths. Small objects should be kept out of their reach to prevent choking.

Play and sleeping areas should be kept free of small objects such as buttons, beads, coins, seeds and nuts.

Very young children should not be given groundnuts (peanuts), hard sweets, or food with small bones or seeds.

Young children should always be supervised during meals. Cut or tear children's food into small pieces.

Coughing, gagging and high-pitched, noisy breathing or the inability to make any sound at all indicate breathing difficulty and possible choking. Choking is a life-threatening emergency. Caregivers should suspect an infant is choking when he or she suddenly has trouble breathing, even if no one has seen the child put something into the mouth. (*See First Aid for Choking, page 140.*)

6.
Poisons, medicines, bleach, acid, and liquid fuels such as paraffin (kerosene) should never be stored in drinking bottles. All such liquids and poisons should be kept in clearly marked containers out of children's sight and reach.

Poisoning is a serious danger to small children. Bleach, insect and rat poison, paraffin (kerosene) and household detergents can kill or permanently injure a child.

Many poisons do not need to be swallowed to be dangerous. They can kill, cause brain damage, blind or permanently injure if they:

- are inhaled
- get onto the child's skin or into the eyes
- get onto the child's clothes.

If poisons are put in soft drink or beer bottles, jars or cups, children may drink them by mistake. All medicines, chemicals and poisons should be stored in their original containers, tightly sealed.

Detergents, bleaches, chemicals and medicines should never be left where children can reach them. They should be tightly sealed and labelled. They should also be locked in a cupboard or trunk or put on a high shelf where children cannot see or reach them.

Medicines meant for adults can kill small children. Medicine should only be given to a child if it was prescribed for that child and never be given to a child if it was prescribed for an adult or some other child.

Overuse or misuse of antibiotics can cause deafness in small children. Medication should only be used as prescribed by the health worker.

Aspirin is a common cause of accidental poisoning. It should be kept out of the reach and sight of children.

7. Children can drown in less than two minutes and in a very small amount of water. They should never be left alone when they are in or near water.

Wells, tubs and buckets of water should be covered.

Children should be taught to swim when they are young as they will then be less likely to drown.

Children should be taught never to swim in fast-flowing streams and never to swim alone.

8. Children under five years old are particularly at risk on the roads. They should always have someone with them and they should be taught safe road behaviour as soon as they can walk.

Young children do not think before they run onto the road. Families need to watch them carefully.

Children should not play near the road, particularly if they are playing with balls.

Children should be taught to walk on the side of the road, facing traffic.

When crossing the road, young children should be taught to:

- stop at the side of the road
- look both ways
- listen for cars or other vehicles before crossing
- hold the hand of another person
- walk, not run.

Older children should be encouraged to look after younger children and to set a good example.

Bicycle accidents are a frequent cause of injury and death among older children. Families can prevent bicycle accidents if they make sure that children with bicycles are trained in road safety. Children should wear helmets or protective headgear when biking.

Children are at high risk of serious injury if they travel in the front seat of a car or unsupervised on the bed of a truck.

INJURY PREVENTION

<table>
<tr><td>✚</td><td># First Aid Advice</td></tr>
</table>

	These first aid measures should be taken to prevent worsening of the situation if medical help is not immediately available.
First aid for burns:	▶ If the child's clothing catches fire, quickly wrap the child in a blanket or clothing or roll her or him on the ground to put out the fire.
	▶ Cool the burned area immediately. Use plenty of cold, clean water. If the burn is extensive, put the child in a bath or basin of cold water. It may take up to half an hour to cool the burned area.
	▶ Keep the burned area clean and dry and protect it with a loose bandage. If the burn is bigger than a large coin or it begins to blister, take the child to a health worker. Do not break the blisters, as they protect the injured area.
	▶ Do not remove anything that is sticking to the burn. Do not put anything except cold water on the burn.
	▶ Give the child fluids such as fruit juice or water with a little sugar and salt.
First aid for electric shocks:	▶ If the child has had an electric shock or burn, turn off the power before touching the child. If the child is unconscious, keep her or him warm and get medical help immediately.
	▶ If the child is having difficulty breathing or is not breathing, lie the child flat on the back and tilt her or his head back slightly. Hold the child's nostrils closed and blow into the mouth. Blow hard enough to make the child's chest rise. Count to three and blow again. Continue until the child begins breathing.

	First Aid Advice
First aid for falls or road injuries:	▶ Injuries to the head and spine, especially the neck, are very dangerous because they can cause lifelong paralysis or be life-threatening. Limit movement of the head and back and avoid any twisting of the spine to prevent further injury. ▶ A child who is unable to move or is in extreme pain may have broken bones. Do not move the injured area. Steady and support it and get medical help immediately. ▶ If the child is unconscious, keep her or him warm and get medical help immediately. ▶ For bad bruises and sprains, immerse the injured area in cold water or put ice on the injury for 15 minutes. Do not put the ice directly on the skin; instead, use a layer of cloth between the ice and the skin. Remove the ice or water, wait 15 minutes and repeat if necessary. The cold should help reduce pain, swelling and bruising.
First aid for cuts and wounds:	**For minor cuts and wounds:** ▶ Wash the wound with very clean (or boiled and cooled) water and soap. ▶ Dry the skin around the wound. ▶ Cover the wound with a clean cloth and place a bandage over it. **For serious cuts and wounds:** ▶ If a piece of glass or other object is sticking in the wound, do not remove it. It may be preventing further bleeding and removing it could make the injury worse. ▶ If the child is bleeding heavily, raise the injured area above the level of the chest and press firmly against the wound (or near it if something is stuck in it) with a pad made of folded clean cloth. Maintain pressure until the bleeding stops. ▶ Do not put any plant or animal matter on the wound, as this could cause infection.

INJURY PREVENTION

	First Aid Advice
First aid for cuts and wounds (continued):	▶ Put a bandage on the wound. Allow for swelling by not tying the bandage too tightly. ▶ Take the child to the health centre or get medical help immediately. Ask the health worker if the child should have a tetanus injection.
First aid for choking:	▶ If an infant or child is coughing, do not interfere – let her or him try to cough up the object. If the object does not release quickly, try to remove the object from the child's mouth. ▶ If the object is still lodged in the child's throat: **For infants or small children:** Support the head and neck. Turn the baby face down with the head lower than the feet. Deliver five blows to the back between the shoulder blades. Turn the baby face up and press firmly on the breastbone between the nipples five times. Repeat until the object is dislodged. If you cannot dislodge the object, take the child to the nearest health worker immediately. **For larger children:** Stand behind the child with your arms around the child's waist. Form a clenched fist with your thumb against the child's body above the navel and below the rib cage. Put the other hand over the fist and give a sharp inward and upward thrust into the child's abdomen. Repeat until the object is dislodged. If you cannot dislodge the object, take the child to the nearest health worker immediately.

	First Aid Advice
First aid for breathing problems or drowning:	▶ If there is any possibility that the head or neck is injured, do not move the child's head. Follow the directions below without moving the head. ▶ If the child is having difficulty breathing or is not breathing, lie the child flat on the back and tilt her or his head back slightly. Hold the child's nostrils closed and blow into the mouth. Blow hard enough to make the child's chest rise. Count to three and blow again. Continue until the child begins breathing. ▶ If the child is breathing but unconscious, roll the child onto her or his side so that the tongue does not block breathing.
First aid for poisoning:	▶ If a child has swallowed poison, do not try to make the child vomit as this may make the child more ill. ▶ If poison is on the child's skin or clothes, remove the clothing and pour large amounts of water over the skin. Wash the skin thoroughly several times with soap. ▶ If a child gets poison in her or his eyes, splash clean water in the eyes for at least 10 minutes. ▶ Take the child immediately to a health centre or hospital. If possible, bring a sample of the poison or medicine or its container with you. Keep the child as still and quiet as possible.

INJURY PREVENTION

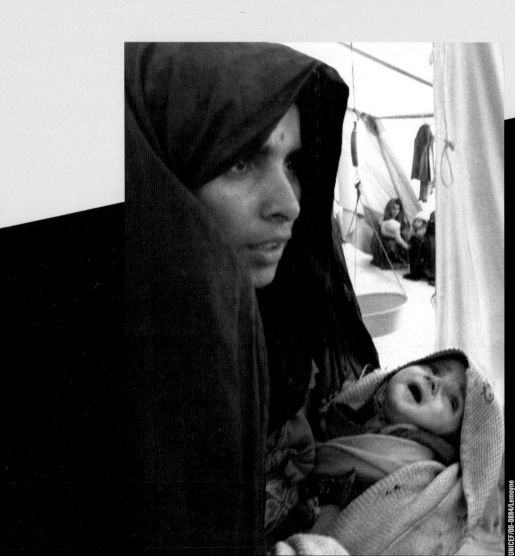

Why it is important to share and act on information about

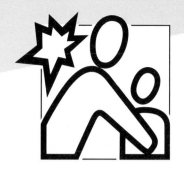

Disasters and Emergencies

In disaster or emergency situations, children are very vulnerable to illness and trauma and require special care and attention.

Of the world's estimated 27 million refugees and 30 million displaced people, 80 per cent are women and children. Almost 2 billion people were affected by disasters from 1990 to 1999. Disasters disproportionately affect the poor. More than 90 per cent of disaster-related deaths occur in developing countries.

Some 9 million children worldwide have been killed, injured, orphaned or separated from their parents by conflicts in the past decade.

Key Messages:

Disasters and Emergencies

1. In disaster or emergency situations, children should receive essential health care, including measles vaccination, adequate food and micronutrient supplements.

2. Breastfeeding is particularly important in emergency situations.

3. It is always preferable for children to be cared for by their parents or other familiar adults, especially during conflict situations, because it makes children feel more secure.

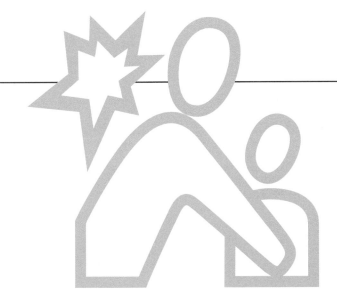

4. Violence in the home, war and other disasters can frighten and anger children. When such events occur, children need special attention, extra affection and the opportunity to express their feelings and to describe their experiences in ways that are appropriate for their age.

5. Landmines and unexploded ammunition are extremely dangerous. They should never be touched or stepped over. Establish safe play areas for children and warn them not to play with unknown objects.

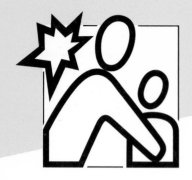

Supporting Information

Disasters and Emergencies

1. In disaster or emergency situations, children should receive essential health care, including measles vaccination, adequate food and micronutrient supplements.

Disease can spread quickly when people are crowded together. All children living in congested conditions, particularly in refugee or disaster situations, should be immunized immediately, especially against measles, at the first point of contact or settlement. Vitamin A supplements should also be provided.

All immunizations in emergency settings should be given with auto-disable syringes – syringes that can be used only once.

Measles is even more serious when children are malnourished or living in conditions of poor sanitation.

● As measles spreads very quickly, a child with measles needs to be isolated from other children, examined by a trained health worker and given vitamin A supplements.

● Measles frequently causes severe diarrhoea. Immunizing children against measles prevents diarrhoea and protects against pneumonia.

If, for any reason, a child has not had the full series of immunizations in the first year of life, it is extremely important to have the child fully immunized as soon as possible.

2. Breastfeeding is particularly important in emergency situations.

Family members, other mothers and skilled health workers are important sources of knowledge and practical support for breastfeeding mothers, to encourage six months of exclusive breastfeeding and continued breastfeeding for two years or beyond. In addition to breastmilk, adequate complementary foods should be provided to children older than six months.

Special attention and support are needed for mothers with stress reactions to overcome the unfounded belief that stress permanently affects breastfeeding.

Special attention to exclusive breastfeeding of babies under six months should be a priority to avoid illness and deaths.

If infant formula is judged to be necessary, the mothers or caregivers involved should have practical counselling on hygienic preparation of feeds. Artificially fed babies need a lot of cuddling and holding. They should never be left alone while self-feeding from a bottle. Cup feeding is recommended.

3. It is always preferable for children to be cared for by their parents or other familiar adults, especially during conflict situations, because it makes children feel more secure.

In crisis or emergency situations, it is the duty of the government, the authorities in charge or the United Nations (in the absence of a government) to ensure that children are not separated from their parents or caregivers.

If separation occurs, it is the responsibility of the government and the authorities in charge to provide special protection and care for the child. The government and the authorities are also responsible for attempting to trace the child's family and for reuniting the child with his or her family.

In emergency situations, interim care must be provided for children who have become separated from their families. Where possible this interim care should be provided by families from the child's community until the child is reunited with relatives or placed with a foster family.

DISASTERS AND EMERGENCIES

FACTS FOR LIFE 147

Children who have become separated from their parents in an emergency situation cannot be assumed to be orphans and are not available for adoption. As long as the fate of a child's parents and/or other close relatives cannot be determined, each separated child must be considered as still potentially having close relatives who are alive. If the parents or relatives cannot be traced, it is best for the child to be adopted by a family of the same origin. Only if that is not possible should adoption by a family from another culture or country be considered.

A move to a new home or country is stressful, especially if the family has fled violence. Refugee children sometimes face the additional burden of having to learn a new language and culture.

4. Violence in the home, war and other disasters can frighten and anger children. When such events occur, children need special attention, extra affection and the opportunity to express their feelings and to describe their experiences in ways that are appropriate for their age.

When familiar people, places or things are lost or threatened, and when adults are too upset or distracted to notice, children may feel afraid and forgotten.

In crisis and emergency situations, parents may find it difficult to give their children affection and security.

It is normal for children to show stress reactions or problem behaviour after frightening, painful or violent experiences. Some children withdraw; others become more aggressive. Some children appear to be coping well, even though they have not worked through their fears. Children may become 'accustomed' to longstanding violence, but it still hurts them.

If children do not receive help to understand their feelings, they may become more upset.

- Regular routines – going to school and maintaining regular eating and sleeping schedules – give children a sense of security and continuity.

- Enjoyable activities help children deal with stress. Opportunities should be created for organized non-violent play, sports and other forms of recreation, such as safe play areas in refugee camps or settlements, to encourage communication and interaction among peers. Drawing or playing with toys or puppets can help children express their feelings and adjust to stressful experiences. Re-enacting stressful situations through play is extremely common and helpful for very young children. This is the child's way of trying to master the impact of what happened.

- Children should be encouraged to talk about what is troubling them. They should be encouraged to express themselves but they must not be forced. They need to be listened to and to express what they have seen or experienced.

- Children between the ages of three and six years may feel responsible for the problem. These feelings may create a strong sense of guilt. These children need support and attention from a caring adult.

- Children need constant reassurance; they should not be scolded or punished. If a close family member has to be away, the child should be told beforehand. The child should be told where the person is going, when he or she will return and who will be caring for the child during the absence.

- Because adolescents have a clearer understanding of war and other traumatic situations, they are in some ways more vulnerable to stressful experiences than younger children and may feel guilt for not being able to prevent the event. They may appear to be coping, but they lack the emotional maturity to deal with traumatic experiences. Adolescents sometimes become aggressive to cope with feelings of anger and depression. They may rebel against authority, use drugs or steal. Or they may withdraw, become fearful or anticipate bad experiences. Adolescents need the help of adults to work through their experiences. Involving adolescents in the life of the community and giving them a role to play is very beneficial.

● Peers, teachers and community members are an important source of support and security for adolescents, who tend to rely less on their immediate families. Adolescents should be encouraged to talk about their experiences with peers and trusted adults and to participate in healing community activities.

● When children's stress reactions are severe and last for a long time, they need special help from a counsellor.

5. Landmines and unexploded ammunition are extremely dangerous. They should never be touched or stepped over. Establish safe play areas for children and warn them not to play with unknown objects.

Landmines come in many different shapes, sizes and colours. Mines can be buried underground or hidden in grass, trees or water. Rusty mines that have been exposed to the weather may be difficult to recognize but they are still dangerous.

Landmines are usually not visible. Special caution is needed near areas of military action or abandoned or overgrown areas. Mined areas may be marked with a picture of a skull and crossbones, crossed sticks or knotted grass. No one should go into these marked areas.

Mines and unexploded ammunition should never be touched. Many of these items are intended to explode when they hit the ground, but sometimes they do not detonate. They are still extremely dangerous. Burning of fields will neither detonate all landmines nor render the area safe.

Some mines are set off by weight, others by tripping or pulling a wire, others just by touching or tilting them. No one should ever step over a trip wire – underground mines may be nearby. Where there is one mine, often there are others. Anyone who sees a mine should stop walking and retrace her or his steps, or stay very still and call for help.

If a landmine injury occurs:

- Apply firm pressure to the bleeding area until the bleeding stops.

- If the bleeding does not seem to be lessening, tie a cloth or piece of clothing (a tourniquet) just above or as close to the wound as possible and send for medical assistance. If help is delayed more than one hour, loosen the tourniquet each hour to check the bleeding. Remove the tourniquet if the bleeding has stopped.

- If the child is breathing but unconscious, roll the child onto her or his side so that the tongue does not block breathing.

Professional demining is the best solution to ensure that the area is safe.

DISASTERS AND EMERGENCIES

Glossary

AIDS	acquired immune deficiency syndrome
BCG	anti-tuberculosis vaccine
DPT	diphtheria/pertussis (whooping cough)/tetanus vaccine
Hib	*Haemophilus influenzae* type B
HIV	human immunodeficiency virus
NGO	non-governmental organization
ORS	oral rehydration salts
PSA	public service announcement
STI	sexually transmitted infection
UNAIDS	Joint United Nations Programme on HIV/AIDS
UNDP	United Nations Development Programme
UNESCO	United Nations Educational, Scientific and Cultural Organization
UNFPA	United Nations Population Fund
UNICEF	United Nations Children's Fund
WFP	World Food Programme
WHO	World Health Organization

Facts for Life Order Form (please send by mail or fax)

I would like to order the following titles:

QUANTITY	SALES NUMBER	TITLE	PRICE IN US$
	E.00.XX.2	**Facts for Life**	$7.50
	F.00.XX.2	**Savoir pour Sauver**	$7.50
	S.00.XX.2	**Para la Vida**	$7.50
		Shipping & Handling	
		TOTAL COST	

POSTAGE AND HANDLING:

Domestic: add 5%, US$5.00 minimum.

Overseas: US$5.00 per copy plus US$5.00 handling charge.

Contact us for **Express Delivery** options.

Payment Information:

Prepayment is required except for UN account holders.

❑ Check/Money Order Enclosed (Payable to "UN Publications" in US$)
   Orders paid by check will be held for 10 days or until the check clears.
   Use of a Credit Card will expedite your order.

❑ Bill my United Nations Account No. _____

Charge my Credit Card: ❑ Visa ❑ MasterCard ❑ American Express

Account # ⬚⬚⬚⬚ ⬚⬚⬚⬚ ⬚⬚⬚⬚ ⬚⬚⬚⬚   Exp. Date ⬚⬚

Signature: _____

Ship to:

Name: _____

Institution: _____

Street Address: _____

City: _____ State: _____ Zip: _____ Country: _____

Telephone: _____ Fax No: _____ E-mail: _____

Submit your order:

In North America, Latin America and the Caribbean and Asia and the Pacific:

United Nations Publications
Sales and Marketing Section
Room DC2-853, Dept. I004
New York, NY 10017, USA
Tel: 1-212-963-8302, 1-800-253-9646
Fax: 1-212-963-3489
E-mail: publications@un.org
Website: www.un.org/Publications

In Europe, Africa and the Middle East:

United Nations Publications
Sales Office and Bookshop
CH-1211 Geneva 10, Switzerland
Tel: 41-22-917-2613, 41-22-917-2614
Fax: 41-22-917-0027
E-mail: unpubli@unog.ch

Visit the UNICEF website to find out about other UNICEF publications:
www.unicef.org/infores/index.html

For further information contact:

United Nations Children's Fund (UNICEF)
Division of Communication
3 UN Plaza, New York, NY 10017, USA
Tel: 1-212-326-7000; Fax: 1-212-303-7985
E-mail: pubdoc@unicef.org Website: www.unicef.org

World Health Organization (WHO)
Avenue Appia 20
CH-1211 Geneva 27, Switzerland
Tel: 41-22-791-2111; Fax: 41-22-791-3111
E-mail: info@who.int Website: www.who.int

**United Nations Educational,
Scientific and Cultural Organization (UNESCO)**
UNESCO House
7, place de Fontenoy
75352 Paris 07 SP, France
Tel: 33-1-4568-1000; Fax: 33-1-4567-1690
E-mail: culture.doc@unesco.org Website: www.unesco.org

United Nations Population Fund (UNFPA)
220 East 42nd Street
New York, NY 10017-5880, USA
Tel: 1-212-297-5026; Fax: 1-212-370-0201
E-mail: HQ@unfpa.org Website: www.unfpa.org

United Nations Development Programme (UNDP)
1 United Nations Plaza
New York, NY 10017, USA
Tel: 1-212-906-5000; Fax: 1-212-906-5364
E-mail: HQ@undp.org Website: www.undp.org

Joint United Nations Programme on HIV/AIDS (UNAIDS)
20, avenue Appia
CH-1211 Geneva 27, Switzerland
Tel: 41-22-791-3666; Fax: 41-22-791-4187
E-mail: unaids@unaids.org Website: www.unaids.org

World Food Programme (WFP)
Via Cesare Giulio Viola 68
Parco dei Medici
00148 Rome, Italy
Tel: 39-06-65131; Fax: 39-06-6513-2840
E-mail: wfpinfo@wfp.org Website: www.wfp.org

The World Bank
1818 H Street, N.W.
Washington, DC 20433, USA
Tel: 1-202-477-1234; Fax: 1-202-477-6391
E-mail: askus@worldbank.org Website: www.worldbank.org